Rapid Clinical Pharmacology

A Student Formulary

D1330235

Rapid Clinical Pharmacology

A Student Formulary

Andrew Batchelder MBChB (Hons), BSc (Hons)
Core Trainee in Surgery
University Hospitals of Leicester NHS Trust
Leicester, UK

Charlene Rodrigues MBChB (Hons), BSc (Hons)
Academic Clinical Fellow in Paediatric Infectious Diseases
Imperial College London
London, UK

Ziad Alrifai MBChB (Hons), MPharm (Hons), MPharmS
Core Trainee in Anaesthetics
University Hospitals of Nottingham NHS Trust
Nottingham, UK

EDITORIAL SUPERVISOR

Adrian G. Stanley PhD, FRCP
Consultant Physician in Cardiovascular Medicine and Honorary Senior Lecturer
(Medical Education)
University Hospitals of Leicester NHS Trust
Leicester, UK

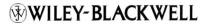

WILEY-BLACKWELL
A John Wiley & Sons, Ltd., Publication

This edition first published 2011 © 2011 by John Wiley and Sons, Ltd

Wiley-Blackwell is an imprint of John Wiley & Sons, formed by the merger of
Wileys global Scientific, Technical and Medical business with Blackwell Publishing.

Registered office: John Wiley & Sons, Ltd, The Atrium, Southern Gate, Chichester, West Sussex,
PO19 8SQ, UK

Editorial offices: 9600 Garsington Road, Oxford, OX4 2DQ, UK
The Atrium, Southern Gate, Chichester, West Sussex, PO19 8SQ, UK
111 River Street, Hoboken, NJ 07030-5774, USA

For details of our global editorial offices, for customer services and for information about how to
apply for permission to reuse the copyright material in this book please see our website
at www.wiley.com/wiley-blackwell

The right of the author to be identified as the author of this work has been asserted in accordance
with the UK Copyright, Designs and Patents Act 1988.

Library of Congress Cataloging-in-Publication Data

Rapid clinical pharmacology : a student formulary / Andrew Batchelder . . . [et al.]. – 1st ed.
      p. ; cm. – (Rapid series)
   Includes index.
   ISBN 978-0-4706-5441-5 (pbk. : alk. paper)
  1. Clinical pharmacology–Handbooks, manuals, etc.   I. Batchelder, Andrew.
II. Series: Rapid series.
   [DNLM: 1. Pharmacology, Clinical–methods–Handbooks.   2. Pharmaceutical
Preparations–administration & dosage–Handbooks.   QV 39]
   RM301.28.R37 2011
   615'.1–dc22

                                                                        2011007199

A catalogue record for this book is available from the British Library.

Set in 7.5/9.5pt, Frutiger-Light by Thomson Digital, Noida, India
Printed and bound in Malaysia by Vivar Printing Sdn Bhd

1   2011

Contents

Central nervous system

Infections

Endocrine system

Obstetrics, gynaecology and urinary tract disorders

Malignant disease and immunosuppression

Musculoskeletal and joint diseases

Eye

Anaesthesia

Intravenous fluids

Blood and transfusion medicine

Preface

In light of the growing pressures on prescribers, increasing emphasis has been placed on the importance of pharmacology in the undergraduate medical curriculum. Clinical pharmacology is a topic with which many students and clinicians struggle because of the large volumes of factual information that they are required to assimilate. In addition, medical students frequently have difficulty identifying the core learning material.

The British Pharmacological Society has recommended that learning be focused on a core list of commonly used drugs and suggests that students create a personal formulary. *Rapid Clinical Pharmacology* provides a concise structured approach for readers, be they students preparing for pharmacology examinations, junior doctors starting out in clinical practice or members of allied health professions involved in prescribing and dispensing medications. The familiar format of the Rapid series emphasises the key headings for each drug class, directing readers to the main points. Special considerations are also given under the 'Important points' heading to highlight features unique to certain drugs or classes.

Good prescribing practice requires knowing which drug to use and why; however, it also requires consideration of comorbidities, potential adverse effects and polypharmacy. Emphasising clinically relevant information about the most commonly used medications, this book provides a good foundation of pharmacological knowledge upon which to build. Additionally, it includes useful tips on prescribing in the context of intravenous fluids and blood components.

We would like to thank Dr Adrian Stanley for the wealth of time and effort he has dedicated to editing this text; without his invaluable assistance this book would not have been possible.

Andrew Batchelder
Charlene Rodrigues
Ziad Alrifai

List of abbreviations

5-HT	5-hydroxytryptamine (serotonin)
ACEIs	Angiotensin-converting enzyme inhibitors
ACh	Acetylcholine
ACS	Acute coronary syndrome
ADH	Antidiuretic hormone
ADP	Adenosine diphosphate
AF	Atrial fibrillation
AIDS	Acquired immunodeficiency syndrome
APTT	Activated partial thromboplastin time
ARBs	Angiotensin receptor blockers
ASA	Aminosalicylic acid
ATP	Adenosine triphosphate
AV	Atrioventricular
AVNRT	AV nodal re-entry tachycardia
BM	Boehringer Mannheim (finger-prick blood glucose)
BP	Blood pressure
BTS	British Thoracic Society
Ca^{2+}	Calcium ion
cAMP	Cyclic adenosine monophosphate
CCBs	Calcium channel blockers
CCF	Congestive cardiac failure
$CD4^+$	Cluster of differentiation 4
cGMP	Cyclic guanosine monophosphate
Cl^-	Chloride ion
CMV	Cytomegalovirus
CNS	Central nervous system
CO_2	Carbon dioxide
COCP	Combined oral contraceptive pill
COMT	Catechol-O-methyl transferase
COPD	Chronic obstructive pulmonary disease
COX	Cyclo-oxygenase
CSF	Cerebrospinal fluid
CT	Computed tomography
CTG	Cardiotocography
CTZ	Chemoreceptor trigger zone
CVP	Central venous pressure
DIC	Disseminated intravascular coagulation
DKA	Diabetic ketoacidosis
DNA	Deoxyribonucleic acid
DVT	Deep vein thrombosis
EBV	Epstein Barr virus
ECG	Electrocardiography
ESR	Erythrocyte sedimentation rate
FBC	Full blood count
FFP	Fresh frozen plasma
FSH	Follicule-stimulating hormone
G6PD	Glucose-6-phosphate dehydrogenase deficiency
GABA	Gamma aminobutyric acid
GFR	Glomerular filtration rate
GI	Gastrointestinal

GLUT	Glucose transporters
GnRH	Gonadotrophin-releasing hormone
GPIIb/IIIa	Glycoprotein IIb/IIIa
GTN	Glyceryl trinitrat
GTP	Guanosine triphosphate
GU	Genito-urinary
H^+	Hydrogen ion
H_1	Histamine type 1 receptor
H_2	Histamine type 2 receptor
HDL	High density lipoproteins
HER2	Human epidermal growth factor receptor 2
HIV	Human immunodeficiency virus
HMG CoA	3-hydroxy-3-methylglutaryl coenzyme A
HONK	Hyperosmolar non-ketotic state
HRT	Hormone replacement therapy
IHD	Ischaemic heart disease
IN	Intranasal
INR	International normalised ratio
ISMN	Isosorbide mononitrate
JVP	Jugular venous pressure
K^+	Potassium ion
L-dopa	Levodopa
LDL	Low-density lipoproteins
LFTs	Liver function tests
LH	Luteinising hormone
LMWH	Low molecular weight heparin
LRTI	Lower respiratory tract infection
LV	Left ventricular
LVF	Left ventricular failure
M_2	Muscarinic type 2 receptors
M_3	Muscarinic type 3 receptors
MAO	Monoamine oxidase
MAOIs	Monoamine oxidase inhibitors
MI	Myocardial infarction
MMSE	Mini-mental state examination
mRNA	Messenger ribonucleic acid
N_2O	Nitrous oxide
Na^+	Sodium ion
NICE	National Institute for Health and Clinical Excellence
NMDA	N-methyl-D-aspartic acid
NNRTIs	Non-nucleoside reverse transcriptase inhibitors
NRTIs	Nucleoside reverse transcriptase inhibitors
NSAID	Non-steroidal anti-inflammatory drugs
O_2	Oxygen
OCP	Oral contraceptive pill
PCA	Patient-controlled analgesia
PCOS	Polycystic ovarian syndrome
PE	Pulmonary embolism
PGs	Prostaglandins
PIs	Protease inhibitors
PO	By mouth (*per os*)
POP	Progesterone-only pill
PONV	Post-operative nausea and vomiting
PPAR	Peroxisome proliferator-activated receptors

PPI	Proton pump inhibitor
PR	Per rectum
PSA	Prostate-specific antigen
QTc	Corrected QT interval
RNA	Ribonucleic acid
SA	Sino-atrial
SERM	Selective oestrogen receptor modulator
SLE	Systemic lupus erythematosus
SNRIs	Serotonin and noradrenaline reuptake inhibitors
SSRIs	Selective serotonin reuptake inhibitors
SVT	Supraventricular tachycardia
$t_{1/2}$	Half-life
T3	Tri-iodothyronine
T4	Tetra-iodothyronine
TCAs	Tricyclic antidepressants
TFTs	Thyroid function tests
TIA	Transient ischaemic attack
TPR	Total peripheral resistance
tRNA	Transfer ribonucleic acid
TSH	Thyroid-stimulating hormone
U&Es	Urea and electrolytes
UTI	Urinary tract infection
VF	Ventricular fibrillation
VLDL	Very low-density lipoproteins
VT	Ventricular tachycardia
VTE	Venous thromboembolism

Abbreviations of routes of administration

IM	Intramuscular
IN	Intranasal
INH	Inhaled
IV	Intravenous
NEB	Nebulised
PO	Oral
PR	Per rectum
PV	Per vagina
SC	Subcutaneous
SL	Sublingual
TOP	Topical

Abbreviations of dosing

OD	Once daily
OM	Once in the morning
ON	Once at night
BD	Twice daily
TDS	Three times a day
QDS	Four times a day
PRN	As required

Basic pharmacokinetic concepts

PHARMACOKINETICS The study of the movement of drugs into, within and out of the body. The key pharmacokinetic parameters from a dosing point of view are bioavailability (F), clearance (Cl), volume of distribution (V_d) and elimination half-life ($t_{1/2}$).

PHARMACODYNAMICS The study of the effect of a drug on the body.

BIOAVAILABILITY (F)

F is defined as the percentage of an administered dose that reaches the systemic circulation unchanged. Bioavailability is 100% for the intravenous route.

Oral bioavailability varies and is dependent on the degree of absorption, formulation of some drugs (e.g. nitrates) and the degree of first-pass hepatic metabolism. If plasma concentration is plotted against time, bioavailability is represented as the area under the curve.

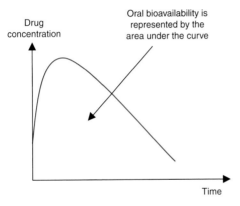

VOLUME OF DISTRIBUTION (V_d)

V_d represents the theoretical volume into which a given drug dose must be distributed in the body to achieve a concentration equal to that of plasma. Drugs that are highly lipid soluble, such as digoxin, have a high V_d. Drugs that are lipid insoluble, such as neuromuscular blockers, remain predominantly in the plasma and will have a low V_d.

Clinically, the larger the volume of distribution the longer it will take to reach a therapeutic level and, therefore, a loading dose may be necessary. The volume of distribution can be calculated as:

$$V_d = \frac{\text{Total amount of drug in body}}{\text{Plasma concentration of drug}}$$

LOADING DOSE

Defined as the initial dose of a drug required to rapidly achieve a desired plasma concentration. The time required to achieve a steady state plasma concentration will be long if a drug has a long $t_{1/2}$ (time taken to reach steady state is approximately 4½ half-lives). Therefore it is desirable to administer a loading dose to attain a therapeutic plasma concentration immediately. Examples of drugs requiring a loading dose regime include amiodarone, digoxin and warfarin.

The main factor determining a loading dose is the volume of distribution (V_d). In order for a drug to reach a steady state plasma concentration (C_p), the tissues into which the drug distributes must be saturated first. The relationship between loading dose and volume of distribution is defined below:

$$\text{Loading dose} = V_d \times C_p$$

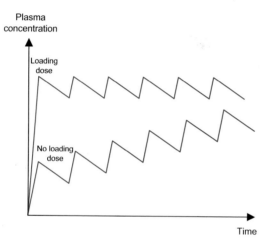

ELIMINATION HALF-LIFE ($t_{1/2}$)

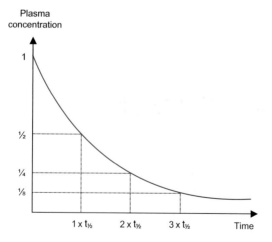

$t_{1/2}$ is the time taken for the plasma concentration of a drug to fall by 50%. The elimination rate constant (K) is the fraction of the total amount of drug in the body removed per unit time. K is represented by the slope of the line of the log plasma concentration versus time.

Elimination rate constant and $t_{1/2}$ can be used clinically to estimate the time to reach steady state concentrations after drug initiation or a change in maintenance dose.

FIRST-ORDER KINETICS

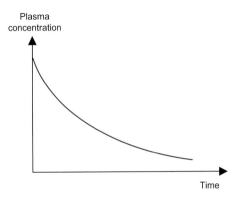

In first-order kinetics a constant fraction of the drug is eliminated per unit time. The rate of elimination is, therefore, proportional to the amount of drug in the body. The majority of drugs follow first-order kinetics.

ZERO-ORDER KINETICS

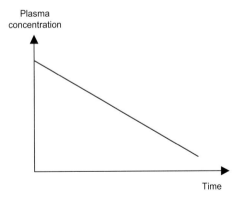

In zero-order kinetics the rate of drug elimination is linear and independent of drug concentration. Many important drugs, such as phenytoin and theophylline, follow zero-order kinetics at higher doses. Alcohol also follows zero-order kinetics with a decline in plasma levels at a constant rate of approximately 15 mg/100 ml/h.

CLEARANCE

Clearance is the theoretical volume of plasma from which the drug is completely removed per unit time. It is not the amount of drug removed from the body. Some of the factors that alter clearance include: degree of protein binding, body surface area, cardiac output, hepatic function and renal function.

Clearance can be calculated from the elimination rate constant and the volume of distribution:

$$Cl = K \times V_d$$

Histamine type 2 receptor antagonists

EXAMPLES   Ranitidine, cimetidine

MECHANISM OF ACTION   Competitive inhibitors of all histamine type 2 receptors. Inhibit histamine- and gastrin-stimulated gastric acid secretion by their action on parietal cells in the stomach.

INDICATIONS
- Gastric and duodenal ulcers
- Gastro-oesophageal reflux
- Treatment and prophylaxis of NSAID-associated ulcers

CAUTIONS AND CONTRA-INDICATIONS
- Hypersensitivity
- If red flag features of malignancy, need to investigate prior to initiating treatment

SIDE-EFFECTS
- GI disturbance, especially diarrhoea
- Gynaecomastia (cimetidine)

METABOLISM AND HALF-LIFE   These drugs are excreted largely unchanged in urine. $t_{1/2}$ is 2–3 h.

MONITORING   No specific drug monitoring required.

DRUG INTERACTIONS
- Cimetidine inhibits Cytochrome P450 activity in the liver and therefore potentiates the action of drugs such as warfarin, phenytoin and theophylline

IMPORTANT POINTS
- Ranitidine can be used prior to general anaesthesia in patients at high risk of aspiration particularly in obstetric practice (Mendelson's syndrome)

Laxatives

MECHANISM OF ACTION

Bulk laxatives (e.g. ispaghula husk) – polysaccharide polymers that are not broken down by digestion and thereby increase stool volume. This stimulates intestinal peristalsis (via the stretch reflex) as well as softening faeces.

Osmotic laxatives (e.g. lactulose, Movicol®) – these poorly absorbed solutes increase the volume of water in the bowel lumen by osmosis hence increasing transit.

Stimulant laxatives (e.g. senna, docusate sodium) – the primary effect is via direct stimulation of myenteric plexus resulting in smooth muscle contraction and increased peristalsis.

Faecal softeners (e.g. arachis oil) – these are surfactants that reduce surface tension and allow water to penetrate and soften faeces.

INDICATIONS
- Constipation
- Hepatic encephalopathy (lactulose)

CAUTIONS AND CONTRA-INDICATIONS
- Bowel obstruction
- Galactosaemia (lactulose only)
- Acute inflammatory bowel disease
- Severe dehydration

SIDE-EFFECTS
- Flatulence
- Diarrhoea
- Abdominal cramps
- Electrolyte disturbances

METABOLISM AND HALF-LIFE   Variable – most are broken down locally in the GI tract with minimal absorption.

MONITORING   No specific drug monitoring required.

DRUG INTERACTIONS
- Lactulose may enhance warfarin effects in severe liver disease

IMPORTANT POINTS
- Before prescribing a laxative ensure constipation is not secondary to an underlying pathology such as bowel cancer
- It requires at least 2–3 days for osmotic or bulking laxatives to take full effect
- Avoid laxatives if bowel obstruction is suspected due to risk of perforation
- Lactulose reduces ammonia-producing organisms and is used in the treatment of hepatic encephalopathy
- Chronic laxative use can cause tolerance (stimulant laxatives)

Proton pump inhibitors (PPIs)

EXAMPLES   Omeprazole, lansoprazole, esomeprazole, pantoprazole

MECHANISM OF ACTION   Inhibit H^+/K^+ ATPase on luminal surface of gastric parietal cells and thereby reduce gastric acid secretion.

INDICATIONS
- Gastric/duodenal ulceration
- As part of triple therapy for eradication of *Helicobacter pylori*
- Gastro-oesophageal reflux disease
- Acid-related dyspepsia
- Hyper-secretory conditions, including Zollinger-Ellison syndrome
- Prevention and treatment of NSAID-associated ulcers

CAUTIONS AND CONTRA-INDICATIONS
- Hypersensitivity
- If red flag features of malignancy need to investigate prior to initiating treatment

SIDE-EFFECTS
- GI disturbance (e.g. abdominal pain, nausea, vomiting, diarrhoea)
- Increased risk of gastric infections due to hypochlorhydria

METABOLISM AND HALF-LIFE   Extensively metabolised by liver and excreted by both renal and biliary routes. $t_{1/2}$ varies from 40 min to 2 h.

MONITORING   No specific drug monitoring required.

DRUG INTERACTIONS
- PPIs are inducers of Cytochrome P450 with some variation in potency between the individual drugs and, therefore, may enhance effects of drugs metabolised by the liver (e.g. phenytoin, carbamazepine, warfarin)

IMPORTANT POINTS
- PPIs reduce acid secretion by >90% and are therefore more effective at healing peptic ulcers than H_2 receptor antagonists (which reduce acid secretion by 50–60%)
- IV PPIs can be used in the management of acute upper GI bleeds under specialist supervision

α-adrenoceptor antagonists (α blockers)

EXAMPLES   Doxazosin, prazosin, tamsulosin, alfuzosin

MECHANISM OF ACTION   Inhibit α_1-adrenoceptors in arterioles, thereby reducing tone of vascular smooth muscle and reducing total peripheral resistance. Inhibition of α_1-adreno-ceptors in periurethral prostatic stroma results in relaxation of internal urethral sphincter and some relief of obstructive urinary symptoms in males.

INDICATIONS
- Hypertension (i.e. doxazosin, particularly in resistant cases as part of polytherapy)
- Benign prostatic hyperplasia

CAUTIONS AND CONTRA-INDICATIONS
- Caution in patients with a susceptibility to heart failure

SIDE-EFFECTS
- Postural hypotension
- Dizziness
- Weakness and fatigue
- Reflex tachycardia
- Headache
- Dry mouth
- Ejaculatory failure

METABOLISM AND HALF-LIFE   Variable – e.g. doxazosin ($t_{1/2}$ ~22 h) extensively metabo-lised by liver; alfuzosin ($t_{1/2}$ ~3–5 h) partially metabolised.

MONITORING   May cause severe first-dose hypotension therefore need to start at low dose and warn patient of side-effects.

DRUG INTERACTIONS
- Enhanced hypotensive effect with antihypertensives and alcohol

IMPORTANT POINTS
- Centrally acting α_2-adrenoceptor agonists (e.g. clonidine, α methyldopa) also have an antihypertensive effect (mediated via suppression of the vasomotor centre in the brain). These agents are rarely used due to infrequent but potentially severe adverse effects (α methyldopa may cause hepatitis). α methyldopa continues to be used for hypertension in pregnancy

Adenosine

MECHANISM OF ACTION   Stimulates specific A1 receptors on the surface of cardiac cells thus influencing adenosine-sensitive K^+ channel and cAMP production. This leads to prolonged conduction through the AV node, often with a high degree AV block.

INDICATIONS
- Rapid reversal of SVT to sinus rhythm
- SVT with aberrant conduction (specialist use only)
- Aiding diagnosis of narrow or broad complex tachycardias

CAUTIONS AND CONTRA-INDICATIONS
- Second and third degree AV block
- Sick sinus syndrome
- Prolonged QT syndrome
- Severe hypotension
- Decompensated heart failure
- Asthma

SIDE-EFFECTS
- Chest pain
- Dyspnoea
- Bronchospasm
- Nausea
- Severe bradycardia
- Choking sensation
- Light-headedness

METABOLISM AND HALF-LIFE $t_{1/2}$ <2 s. Metabolised by uptake into red blood cells and deaminated in plasma.

MONITORING   Cardiac monitoring required.

DRUG INTERACTIONS
- Effects of adenosine are potentiated by dipyridamole

IMPORTANT POINTS
- Ensure patient is linked to a cardiac monitor or defibrillator
- Attempt vasovagal manoeuvres prior to administration unless contra-indicated
- If no response to the above, start with 6 mg IV rapid bolus given through a large vein and flush with 20 ml of normal saline
- Repeat with 12 mg after 1–2 minutes if no response. A further 12 mg can be given
- Early specialist cardiology advice is warranted if no response to 12 mg of adenosine or if adverse signs are present at any stage e.g. heart failure
- Patients should be informed prior to adenosine administration of possible chest pain and the sensation of the heart ceasing to beat

Aldosterone antagonists

EXAMPLES   Spironolactone, eplerenone

MECHANISM OF ACTION   Competitive antagonist at intracellular aldosterone receptors in renal tubules causing reduced production of aldosterone-induced proteins. This indirectly reduces activity of Na^+/K^+ ATPase in the collecting ducts, increasing excretion of Na^+ and decreasing K^+ loss. Spironolactone, in particular, also acts on receptors in other tissues, including androgen receptors.

INDICATIONS
- Congestive cardiac failure (spironolactone)
- Oedema and ascites in liver disease (spironolactone)
- Post-MI heart failure (eplerenone)
- Nephrotic syndrome (spironolactone)
- Primary hyperaldosteronism (including Conn's syndrome) (spironolactone)

CAUTIONS AND CONTRA-INDICATIONS
- Electrolyte disturbances (including hyperkalaemia and hyponatraemia)
- Caution in renal impairment

SIDE-EFFECTS
- Hyperkalaemia (K^+ sparing effect)
- GI disturbance
- Anti-androgenic effects (spironolactone – menstrual irregularities in females, gynaecomastia and hypogonadism in males)

METABOLISM AND HALF-LIFE   Metabolised to active metabolites. $t_{1/2}$ of drug is 60–90 min but $t_{1/2}$ of active metabolites is longer (up to 11 h).

MONITORING   Monitor plasma electrolytes for adverse effects as above.

DRUG INTERACTIONS
- Enhanced hypotensive effect with other antihypertensives
- Increased risk of hyperkalaemia with ACEIs/ARBs and amiloride
- Increased risk of nephrotoxicity with NSAIDs

IMPORTANT POINTS
- Eplerenone is more selective than spironolactone and therefore causes fewer sex hormone-related adverse effects
- Spironolactone may also be used in hypertension (unlicensed indication)

Amiodarone

MECHANISM OF ACTION Inhibits Na^+/K^+ ATPases in myocardium. Prolongs action potential duration and refractory period, slows AV conduction and SA node function.

INDICATIONS
- Paroxysmal SVT
- Nodal and ventricular tachycardias
- Atrial fibrillation and flutter
- VF
- Tachyarrhythmias associated with Wolff–Parkinson–White syndrome

CAUTIONS AND CONTRA-INDICATIONS
- Sinus bradycardia
- SA node block
- Thyroid dysfunction

SIDE-EFFECTS
- Photosensitive rash
- Slate-grey skin discolouration
- Bradycardia
- Hypothyroidism or hyperthyroidism
- Corneal microdeposits (dazzling at night)
- Pulmonary fibrosis/pneumonitis

METABOLISM AND HALF-LIFE Plasma $t_{1/2}$ is long ~50 days (ranges from 10–100 days)

MONITORING LFTs, TFTs and chest x-ray prior to commencing treatment. LFTs and TFTs every 6 months while on treatment.

DRUG INTERACTIONS
- Increases plasma levels of warfarin, digoxin and phenytoin (reduce doses accordingly) leading to toxicity
- Drugs that prolong QT interval

IMPORTANT POINTS
- Should only be initiated under specialist supervision
- ECG monitoring required when given intravenously
- Should be administered through a central line or large IV cannula
- Can cause torsades de pointes, particularly in individuals with prolonged QT interval (congenital or acquired)

Angiotensin-converting enzyme inhibitors (ACEIs)

EXAMPLES   Ramipril, lisinopril, perindopril

MECHANISM OF ACTION   Inhibit angiotensin-converting enzyme, preventing the conversion of angiotensin I to angiotensin II. This prevents angiotensin II-mediated effects (arteriolar constriction and aldosterone release) resulting in reduced afterload and reduced circulating volume, thereby reducing BP.

INDICATIONS
- Hypertension
- Heart failure (result in improved survival in LV dysfunction)
- Prophylaxis of further cardiovascular events post-MI
- Diabetic nephropathy (lisinopril - results in reduced progression of disease)
- Patients at high cardiovascular risk (ramipril)

CAUTIONS AND CONTRA-INDICATIONS
- Hypersensitivity to ACEIs
- Pregnancy
- Renal artery stenosis (reversal of angiotensin II-mediated constriction of efferent arteriole results in reduced GFR)
- Caution in peripheral vascular disease as this may be associated with undiagnosed renal artery stenosis

SIDE-EFFECTS
- Persistent dry cough
- Hypotension (may get severe first-dose hypotension)
- Renal impairment
- Hyperkalaemia
- Angioedema (rare)

METABOLISM AND HALF-LIFE   Variable – e.g. ramipril ($t_{1/2}$ 13–17 h) has an active metabolite; lisinopril ($t_{1/2}$ ~12 h) does not undergo metabolism.

MONITORING   Monitor U&Es for renal impairment prior to and 1–2 weeks after commencing treatment. Once stable on therapy U&Es must be checked at least annually. Careful clinical monitoring is required when used in severe heart failure.

DRUG INTERACTIONS
- Risk of profound first-dose hypotension with loop diuretics and enhanced hypotensive effect with other antihypertensive agents
- Increased risk of renal impairment with NSAIDs
- Enhanced hypoglycaemic effect of insulin, metformin and sulfonylureas
- Effects are antagonised by corticosteroids

IMPORTANT POINTS
- Clinical effects of the different agents are similar; choice determined by $t_{1/2}$ (e.g. lisinopril has longer $t_{1/2}$, therefore suitable for once daily dosing) and by side-effect profile
- ACEIs/ARBs are less effective in African–Caribbean patients due to ACE polymorphisms

Angiotensin II receptor blockers (ARBs)

EXAMPLES Candesartan, losartan, valsartan, irbesartan

MECHANISM OF ACTION Act as antagonists at angiotensin II (type 1) receptors. This prevents angiotensin II-mediated effects (arteriolar constriction and aldosterone release) resulting in reduced afterload and reduced circulating volume, thereby reducing BP.

INDICATIONS
- Hypertension
- Heart failure (result in improved survival in LV dysfunction)
- Diabetic nephropathy in type 2 diabetes

CAUTIONS AND CONTRA-INDICATIONS
- Pregnancy
- Renal artery stenosis (reversal of angiotensin II-mediated constriction of efferent arteriole results in reduced GFR)
- Caution in peripheral vascular disease as this may be associated with undiagnosed renal artery stenosis

SIDE-EFFECTS
- Hypotension (may get severe first-dose hypotension)
- Renal impairment
- Hyperkalaemia
- Angioedema (rare)

METABOLISM AND HALF-LIFE Variable – e.g. valsartan ($t_{1/2}$ 6 h) is excreted largely unchanged via the biliary route; losartan ($t_{1/2}$ of active metabolite is 6–9 h) is excreted via biliary and urinary routes.

MONITORING Monitor U&Es for renal impairment prior to and 1–2 weeks after commencing treatment. Once stable on therapy U&Es must be checked at least annually. Careful clinical monitoring is required when used in severe heart failure.

DRUG INTERACTIONS
- Risk of profound first-dose hypotension with loop diuretics and enhanced hypotensive effect with other antihypertensive agents
- Increased risk of renal impairment with NSAIDs
- Enhanced hypoglycaemic effect of insulin, metformin and sulfonylureas
- Effects are antagonised by corticosteroids

IMPORTANT POINTS
- ACEIs inhibit ACE-mediated break down of bradykinin; bradykinin stimulates vagal afferent nerve fibres and produces a refractory dry cough. This side-effect does not occur with ARBs as they do not act directly on ACE
- ACEIs/ARBs are less effective in African/Caribbean patients due to ACE polymorphisms

Antimuscarinics

EXAMPLES   Atropine, hyoscine, procyclidine

MECHANISM OF ACTION   Antimuscarinics act as competitive antagonists of ACh on effector cells by blocking specific muscarinic receptors (e.g. atropine blocks cardiac M_2 receptors). Their therapeutic action stems mainly from inhibition of smooth muscle contraction and glandular tissue innervated by postganglionic cholinergic neurones.

INDICATIONS
- Bradycardia (atropine)
- Mydriasis and cycloplegia
- Parkinsonism (procyclidine)
- Symptomatic relief of GI or GU muscle spasm (hyoscine)
- Urinary incontinence (see Oxybutynin, p.97)

CAUTIONS AND CONTRA-INDICATIONS
- Myasthenia gravis
- Paralytic ileus
- Pyloric stenosis
- Prostatic enlargement

SIDE-EFFECTS
- Constipation
- Urinary retention
- Dry mouth
- Blurred vision
- Drowsiness

METABOLISM AND HALF-LIFE   Highly variable – $t_{1/2}$ for atropine is 2–4 h and it is metabolised by the liver to inactive metabolites; $t_{1/2}$ for hyoscine is ~5 h; $t_{1/2}$ for procyclidine is ~12 h.

MONITORING   Administration of atropine requires cardiac and blood pressure monitoring.

DRUG INTERACTIONS
- Increased sedative effect when hyoscine given with alcohol

IMPORTANT POINTS
- Hyoscine may be used for GI colic and excessive respiratory secretions in end-of-life care. It is also used to reduce respiratory secretions during anaesthesia
- Atropine is used as part of the Resuscitation Council UK guidelines for symptomatic bradycardia and in cardiac arrests when pulseless electrical activity is below 60 complexes per min

Aspirin

1 2 2

MECHANISM OF ACTION   Irreversibly inhibits cyclo-oxygenase, resulting in reduced platelet aggregation via impaired thromboxane A2 and prostacyclin production within platelets. Inhibition of thromboxane A2 persists for the lifespan of the platelet (7–10 days). Inhibition of prostacyclin is temporary as production by endothelial cells is continuous.

INDICATIONS
- Prophylaxis of MI
- Prophylaxis of cerebrovascular disease
- AF (if warfarin is not indicated)
- Mild to moderate pain
- Pyrexia

CAUTIONS AND CONTRA-INDICATIONS
- Active peptic ulcer
- Haemophilia
- Bleeding diathesis
- Hypersensitivity

SIDE-EFFECTS
- Bronchospasm
- GI and other haemorrhage
- GI disturbance

METABOLISM AND HALF-LIFE   Metabolised by liver; $t_{1/2}$ ~4 h.

MONITORING   No specific drug monitoring required.

DRUG INTERACTIONS
- Use of aspirin and anticoagulants increases the risk of bleeding
- Increased risk of GI side-effects with corticosteroids

IMPORTANT POINTS
- Low dose aspirin (75 mg) used for long-term prophylaxis. High dose (300 mg) is given if an ischaemic event is suspected
- If at high risk of upper GI bleed, give a proton pump inhibitor in conjunction with aspirin
- Can cause Reye's syndrome (hepatic and CNS disorder) in children under 16 years old
- In overdose may cause a respiratory alkalosis (adults) due to hyperventilation and a metabolic acidosis (children) due to salicylate load and accumulation of lactic, pyruvic and aceto-acetic acid

① Low dose Aspirin + heparin ⇒ reduce miscarriages
   * Last 3months, no higher   (↓ blood clots)
        than > 100mg

② Aspirin → breast milk so only take a very low
   dose. 75mg   Reye's syndrome otherwise
   ⇒ Risk of

β-adrenoceptor antagonists (β blockers)

EXAMPLES   Atenolol, propranolol, bisoprolol, carvedilol, sotalol, labetalol, nebivolol

MECHANISM OF ACTION Block activation of β-adrenoceptors (predominantly mediated through β_1 antagonism) thereby reducing exertionally-induced rise in heart rate and reducing cardiac contractility. This reduces systolic BP and myocardial O_2 demand.

INDICATIONS
- Angina
- Arrhythmias
- Hypertension
- Heart failure (bisoprolol and carvedilol only)
- Prophylaxis post-MI
- Migraine prophylaxis
- Thyrotoxicosis
- Anxiety

CAUTIONS AND CONTRA-INDICATIONS
- Asthma
- Uncontrolled heart failure
- Bradycardia, sick sinus syndrome, second or third degree heart block
- Hypotension/cardiogenic shock
- Severe peripheral arterial disease

SIDE-EFFECTS
- Bronchospasm
- Fatigue
- Cold peripheries
- Bradycardia and hypotension
- Sleep disturbances
- Reduced glucose tolerance
- Hyperkalaemia
- Sexual dysfunction in males
- Dizziness and headache
- Heart block

METABOLISM AND HALF-LIFE Variable – e.g. atenolol ($t_{1/2}$ ~6 h) is excreted largely unchanged in urine; propranolol ($t_{1/2}$ ~4 h) is metabolised by the liver.

MONITORING   Monitor clinically for adverse effects.

DRUG INTERACTIONS
- Enhanced hypotensive effects with antihypertensives and alcohol
- Hypotensive effect antagonised by NSAIDs, steroids and oestrogens
- May mask warning signs of hypoglycaemia in diabetics
- Increased risk of AV block and heart failure with verapamil and diltiazem

IMPORTANT POINTS
- Cardioselectivity: atenolol, bisoprolol and nebivolol have less effect on β_2 receptors and therefore reduced bronchospasm
- Lipid solubility: atenolol and sotalol are most water-soluble therefore less able to cross blood–brain barrier resulting in less sleep disturbance
- Half-life: atenolol, bisoprolol and carvedilol have longer duration of action hence only need to be taken once daily

β-adrenoceptor antagonists (β blockers) (continued)

- Additional effects: sotalol is a mixed class II/III antiarrhythmic (requires monitoring of QT interval due to risk of torsades de pointes). Nebivolol causes peripheral vasodilatation (mediated by nitric oxide)
- Intravenous labetolol can be used as a treatment for hypertensive emergencies, particularly those associated with pregnancy

Calcium channel blockers (CCBs)

EXAMPLES Dihydropyridines (nifedipine, amlodipine, felodipine), diltiazem, verapamil

MECHANISM OF ACTION Block L-type Ca^{2+} channels to reduce influx of Ca^{2+} into cells and thereby reduce contraction of myocytes. Dihydropyridines are highly vascular selective and cause peripheral and coronary vasodilatation. Verapamil and diltiazem are less selective and act directly on cardiac tissue to reduce cardiac contractility and slow conduction at the AV node.

INDICATIONS
- Hypertension
- SVT (verapamil and diltiazem)
- Prophylaxis of angina
- Raynaud's phenomenon (dihydropyridines only)
- Cluster headache prophylaxis (verapamil)

CAUTIONS AND CONTRA-INDICATIONS
- Cardiogenic shock or hypotension
- LVF (verapamil and diltiazem)
- Second or third degree heart block (verapamil and diltiazem)
- Bradycardia (verapamil and diltiazem)
- Unstable angina (dihydropyridines)

SIDE-EFFECTS
- Bradycardia (verapamil and diltiazem)
- Reflex tachycardia (dihydropyridines)
- Hypotension
- Vasodilatory effects (flushing, headache, ankle swelling, palpitations)
- Constipation (verapamil)
- Heart failure (verapamil)

METABOLISM AND HALF-LIFE All extensively metabolised in liver. $t_{1/2}$ for diltiazem is 3–5 h; $t_{1/2}$ for verapamil is ~6 hours; $t_{1/2}$ for dihydropyridines is highly variable.

MONITORING No specific drug monitoring required.

DRUG INTERACTIONS
- Enhanced hypotensive effects with antihypertensives and alcohol
- Increased risk of AV block, bradycardia, severe hypotension and heart failure if verapamil or diltiazem are given with β blockers
- Plasma concentration of some CCBs are increased by grapefruit juice

IMPORTANT POINTS
- Verapamil and diltiazem are Vaughan Williams class IV anti-arrhythmics
- Vascular selectivity of different CCBs is explained by voltage dependence; dihydropyridines are inactive at the hyperpolarised membrane potentials of the myocardium during diastole. Verapamil and diltiazem are less voltage dependent and hence less selective

Cardiac glycosides

EXAMPLE Digoxin

MECHANISM OF ACTION Inhibits Na^+/K^+ ATPase in myocardium and thereby reduces extrusion of Ca^{2+}. This prolongs phases 4 and 0 of the cardiac action potential resulting in an increase in end diastolic filling and force of contraction (in accordance with the Frank–Starling law of the heart). Indirectly slows conduction at SA node and AV node and centrally stimulates the vagus nerve, resulting in a negative chronotropic effect.

INDICATIONS
- Supraventricular arrythmias (atrial fibrillation and atrial flutter)
- Heart failure

CAUTIONS AND CONTRA-INDICATIONS
- Complete heart block and second degree block
- Tachyarrhythmias associated with Wolff–Parkinson–White syndrome
- Ventricular tachycardia/fibrillation
- Myocarditis/constrictive pericarditis
- Hypertrophic cardiomyopathy

SIDE-EFFECTS
- GI disturbance
- Dizziness
- Blurred or yellow vision (xanthopsia suggests toxicity)
- Arrhythmias/conduction defects
- Rash
- Abdominal pain (suggests toxicity)

METABOLISM AND HALF-LIFE PLASMA $t_{1/2}$ is ~36 h. Exclusively eliminated by the kidneys, hence need to reduce maintenance dose in elderly patients and in renal impairment.

MONITORING Check U&Es prior to initiation of treatment. Digoxin levels should be taken 6 h post dose.

DRUG INTERACTIONS
- Increased risk of AV block and symptomatic bradycardia with β blockers
- Risk of cardiac toxicity secondary to hypokalaemia with diuretics
- Plasma concentrations increased by verapamil and diltiazem
- Plasma concentration increased by amiodarone and reduced by St John's wort

IMPORTANT POINTS
- Hypokalaemia and hypercalcaemia predispose to digoxin toxicity
- Narrow therapeutic index hence risk of toxicity
- Requires loading dose at initiation of treatment

Clopidogrel

MECHANISM OF ACTION The active metabolite selectively inhibits the binding of ADP to its platelet receptor and the subsequent activation of GPIIb/IIIa complex, inhibiting platelet aggregation.

INDICATIONS
- Acute coronary syndrome
- Acute ST elevation MI
- Aspirin intolerance/hypersensitivity
- Prophylaxis of atherosclerotic events in patients with coronary, cerebral or peripheral vascular disease

CAUTIONS AND CONTRA-INDICATIONS
- Active bleeding (e.g. peptic ulcer, intracranial haemorrhage)

SIDE-EFFECTS
- Bleeding
- GI disturbance
- Gastric and duodenal ulcers

by cP4 50

METABOLISM AND HALF-LIFE Clopidogrel is a prodrug, extensively metabolised in the liver to produce the active metabolite. $t_{1/2}$ of the main metabolite is 8 h.

MONITORING No specific drug monitoring required.

DRUG INTERACTIONS
- Caution if given in combination with other antiplatelet, anticoagulant or fibrinolytics due to risk of bleeding

IMPORTANT POINTS
- Can be given in combination with low-dose aspirin in ACS and acute MI
- Given as loading dose (300–600 mg) at initiation of treatment
- Usually stopped 7 days pre-operatively, to reduce the risk of peri-operative bleeding
- Combination with warfarin (e.g. in patients with AF presenting with ACS) significantly increases the risk of bleeding

* inhibit ADP platelet receptors causing
① Inhibition of the expression of GPIIa/IIb complex
② the complexes are receptors for fibrinogen
→ reduce platelet aggregation

Dipyridamole

MECHANISM OF ACTION Inhibits adenosine deaminase and phosphodiesterase, preventing the degradation of cAMP. This reduces production of thromboxane A2 and platelet activation and aggregation.

INDICATIONS
- Ischaemic stroke and TIA
- Adjunct to warfarin for prophylaxis of thromboembolism with prosthetic heart valves

CAUTIONS AND CONTRA-INDICATIONS
- Hypersensitivity

SIDE-EFFECTS
- GI disturbance
- Worsening coronary heart disease
- Bleeding

METABOLISM AND HALF-LIFE Plasma $t_{1/2}$ is 9–12 h; predominantly excreted in bile.

MONITORING No specific drug monitoring required.

DRUG INTERACTIONS
- Enhances cardiovascular effects of adenosine
- Caution if given in combination of other antiplatelets, anticoagulants or fibrinolytics due to risk of bleeding

IMPORTANT POINTS
- Used in combination with anticoagulation in patients with prosthetic heart valves, and low-dose aspirin in patients with ischaemic stroke/TIA
- Only the modified release formulation is licensed for these indications

Fibrates

EXAMPLES   Fenofibrate, bezafibrate, gemfibrozil

MECHANISM OF ACTION   Increase activity of lipoprotein lipase to facilitate catabolism of VLDL (by promoting entry of triglycerides from VLDL and chylomicrons into target tissues). Fibrates also increase the cholesterol content of HDL particles.

INDICATIONS
- Primary hyperlipidaemia
- Serum triglycerides >10 mmol/l
- Intolerance to statins

CAUTIONS AND CONTRA-INDICATIONS
- Severe hepatic or renal impairment (resulting in low albumin e.g. nephrotic syndrome)
- Primary biliary cirrhosis
- Gallbladder disease

SIDE-EFFECTS
- GI disturbance
- Myositis-like syndrome (uncommon)
- Cholestasis and increased risk of cholelithiasis

METABOLISM AND HALF-LIFE   Variable – e.g. fenofibrate ($t_{1/2}$ ~20 h) is excreted largely unchanged in urine; gemfibrozil ($t_{1/2}$ ~1½ h) is eliminated mainly by metabolism.

MONITORING   Monitor LFTs (especially if concomitant statin use); only measure creatine kinase if clinically indicated.

DRUG INTERACTIONS
- Increased risk of rhabdomyolysis with statins (especially gemfibrozil)
- Enhanced anticoagulant effect of warfarin
- Increased risk of hypoglycaemia with oral antidiabetic agents

IMPORTANT POINTS
- Fibrates may be required in combination with statins in diabetic patients to achieve target lipid lowering

Fibrinolytics

EXAMPLES   Streptokinase, alteplase, reteplase, tenecteplase

MECHANISM OF ACTION   Activation of plasminogen to form plasmin, a proteolytic enzyme that promotes the breakdown of fibrin clots into fibrin degrading products leading to clot dissolution and reperfusion.

INDICATIONS
- Acute MI
- Massive pulmonary embolus (alteplase)
- Acute ischaemic stroke (under specialist supervision by stroke physician)

CAUTIONS AND CONTRA-INDICATIONS
- Aortic dissection
- Active bleeding
- Active peptic ulcer disease
- Previous haemorrhagic stroke or recent ischaemic stroke
- Coagulation defects
- Recent surgery/trauma
- Active intracranial neoplasm
- Uncontrolled hypertension (relative contraindication)

SIDE-EFFECTS
- Bleeding (including cerebral haemorrhage)
- Nausea and vomiting
- Reperfusion cardiac arrhythmias and ischaemia
- Cerebral and pulmonary oedema
- Anaphylaxis
- Severe hypotension

METABOLISM AND HALF-LIFE   Variable – $t_{1/2}$ for streptokinase is 18–23 min; $t_{1/2}$ for alteplase is 4–5 min. Metabolised predominantly by the liver.

MONITORING   Monitor for signs of bleeding, anaphylaxis and intracranial haemorrhage.

DRUG INTERACTIONS
- Risk of haemorrhage is increased with oral anticoagulants
- Patients on ACEIs are at an increased risk of anaphylactoid reaction when streptokinase is administered

IMPORTANT POINTS
- Fibrinolytics are licensed for ST elevation MI within 12 h of the onset of chest pain (administered ideally within one hour)
- Streptokinase is derived from *β-haemolytic Streptococci* of Lancefield group C; persistence of antibodies to streptokinase may reduce the effect of subsequent doses. It has effectively been superseded by the newer fibrinolytics (e.g. reteplase) in acute MI (where primary percutaneous coronary intervention is not available)
- Alteplase is a recombinant tissue-type plasminogen activator. Does not cause allergic reactions and can be used in patients with recent streptococcal infections or recent use of streptokinase

Flecainide

MECHANISM OF ACTION   Vaughan Williams Class Ic antiarrhythmic. Blocks Na^+ dependent channels hence depressing phase 0 of the cardiac action potential. Increased PR and QRS intervals and lengthened ventricular refractory period lead to slower conduction of electrical impulses, with the greatest effect noted on the bundle of His and Purkinje system. In addition to negative chronotropic effect, flecainide also reduces contractility.

INDICATIONS
- Wolff–Parkinson–White syndrome
- AV nodal reciprocating tachycardia (AVNRT)
- Ventricular tachyarrhythmias

CAUTIONS AND CONTRA-INDICATIONS
- Second and third degree AV block
- SA node dysfunction
- Impaired LV function
- Long-standing AF
- History of structural heart disease e.g. previous MI

SIDE-EFFECTS
- Arrhythmia
- Dyspnoea
- Dizziness
- Hypersensitivity
- Oedema
- Fatigue
- Fever
- Visual disturbances

METABOLISM AND HALF-LIFE $t_{1/2}$ is 12–27 h. Predominantly metabolised in the liver to an active metabolite.

MONITORING   Cardiac monitoring is required during intravenous administration.

DRUG INTERACTIONS
- Increased concentrations of flecainide when given with amiodarone
- Risk of myocardial depression and bradycardia with β blockers
- Increased risk of cardiac toxicity when given with diuretics (secondary to hypokalaemia)
- Risk of ventricular arrhythmias when given with tricyclic antidepressants

IMPORTANT POINTS
- Flecainide should be initiated by a specialist
- Bolus dose should only be given in an emergency situation with cardiac monitoring and resuscitation facilities available
- Flecainide demonstrates use-dependence i.e. its effect on Na^+ channels increases with increasing heart rate
- Can be used as a 'pill-in-the-pocket' for self-administration in paroxysmal SVT

Glycoprotein IIb/IIIa inhibitors

EXAMPLES   Tirofiban, eptifibatide

MECHANISM OF ACTION   Non-peptide antagonist that prevents fibrinogen from binding to the glycoprotein IIb/IIIa receptor, thus blocking platelet aggregation.

INDICATIONS
- Unstable angina/non-ST elevation MI (given with aspirin and heparin)
- Reduce the immediate risk of vascular occlusion in patients undergoing percutaneous coronary intervention

CAUTIONS AND CONTRA-INDICATIONS
- Active bleeding
- Major surgery or trauma in past 6 weeks
- Ischaemic stroke within 30 days or any history of haemorrhagic stroke
- Intracranial pathology (e.g. aneurysm, neoplasm or AV malformation)
- Severe hypertension
- Deranged clotting or thrombocytopenia

SIDE-EFFECTS
- Bleeding
- Nausea
- Headaches
- Fever
- Reversible thrombocytopenia

METABOLISM AND HALF-LIFE $t_{1/2}$ of tirofiban is $\sim$90 min. Excreted largely unchanged in urine.

MONITORING   Continuous cardiac monitoring. Monitor clinically for signs of bleeding.

DRUG INTERACTIONS
- Risk of haemorrhage is increased with heparin and antiplatelet drugs

IMPORTANT POINTS
- NICE guidelines recommend tirofiban or eptifibatide for patients at high risk of MI or death when early percutaneous coronary intervention is desirable but not immediately accessible
- Concomitant heparin is a requirement
- Treatment should be for a minimum of 48 h and a maximum of 108 h if the patient remains unstable with a view to in-patient angiography and potential revascularisation as soon as possible

Inotropic sympathomimetics

EXAMPLES   Adrenaline, dopamine, dobutamine, isoprenaline

MECHANISM OF ACTION   Actions vary depending on which receptors are stimulated. Adrenaline acts on α- (peripheral vasculature) and β-adrenoceptors (myocardium), producing positive inotropic and chronotropic effects. Low-dose dopamine and dobutamine stimulate β_1-adrenoceptors in the myocardium, predominantly increasing contractility.

INDICATIONS
- Cardiogenic shock
- Septic shock
- Acute hypotension
- Cardiac arrest (adrenaline)

CAUTIONS AND CONTRA-INDICATIONS
- Phaechromocytoma (dopamine)
- Atrial and ventricular tachyarrhythmias (dobutamine)

SIDE-EFFECTS
- Nausea and vomiting
- Hypotension/hypertension
- Peripheral vasoconstriction
- Tachycardia

METABOLISM AND HALF-LIFE   Metabolised by liver, kidney or plasma MAO and COMT; $t_{1/2}$ $\sim$2 min.

MONITORING   Continuous cardiac monitoring in a high-dependency area is required. Monitoring of oxygen saturation, urine output and renal function is also necessary.

DRUG INTERACTIONS
- Adrenaline should not be used with other sympathomimetic agents due to the additive effect
- Hypertensive crisis when given in combination with MAOIs
- Hypertension and reflex bradycardia when given in combination with β blockers

IMPORTANT POINTS
- In patients with septic or haemorrhagic shock, volume must be replaced (though this may worsen cardiogenic shock), after which sympathomimetics may be required to improve cardiac output
- Often used in the intensive care setting to maintain perfusion to vital organs
- Adrenaline is used as part of the Resuscitation Council UK guidelines

Loop diuretics

EXAMPLES Furosemide, bumetanide

MECHANISM OF ACTION   Inhibits the reabsorption of Na^+ and Cl^- in the ascending limb of the Loop of Henle by inhibiting the $Na^+/K^+/2Cl^-$ co-transporter. This results in increased Na^+ excretion and free water clearance, thereby reducing preload.

INDICATIONS
- Pulmonary oedema secondary to LVF
- Chronic heart failure

CAUTIONS AND CONTRA-INDICATIONS
- Severe hypokalaemia/hyponatraemia
- Hypovalaemia
- Renal failure due to nephrotoxic drugs
- Comatose patients with liver cirrhosis
- Anuria

SIDE-EFFECTS
- Electrolyte disturbances (hypokalaemia, hyponatraemia, hypocalcaemia)
- Hypotension
- Tinnitus and deafness (associated with large IV boluses)
- GI disturbance
- Dyslipidaemia

METABOLISM AND HALF-LIFE $t_{1/2}$ is variable (furosemide ~90 min). Onset of action occurs within 1 h and diuresis is complete within 6 h. Excreted largely unchanged in the urine.

MONITORING   Check U&Es prior to initiating and during treatment.

DRUG INTERACTIONS
- Risk of cardiotoxicity when given with digoxin (secondary to hypokalaemia)
- Risk of ototoxicity when given with aminoglycosides or vancomycin
- Enhanced hypotensive effect with other antihypertensives
- Can reduce lithium excretion
- NSAIDs can reduce effectiveness of loop diuretics (due to reduced GFR)

IMPORTANT POINTS
- Patients with low GFR may require higher doses (diuretic resistance due to poor perfusion to target tissues)
- IV furosemide has very early venodilatory effect

Low molecular weight heparins (LMWH)

EXAMPLES Dalteparin, enoxaparin, tinzaparin

MECHANISM OF ACTION Activate antithrombin III (serine protease inhibitor) thus inhibiting factors IIa (thrombin) and Xa in the common pathway of the clotting cascade. Secondary effects mediated by impairing adhesion and aggregation of platelets.

INDICATIONS
- Prevention of VTE
- Treatment of VTE and acute coronary syndrome/MI
- Prevention of clotting in extracorporeal circuits

CAUTIONS AND CONTRA-INDICATIONS
- Heparin sensitivity
- Haemophilia and other bleeding disorders
- Severe hypertension
- Severe hepatic or renal disease
- In patients undergoing surgery on brain, eye or spinal cord

SIDE-EFFECTS
- Bleeding
- Heparin-induced thrombocytopenia
- Hypersensitivity reaction
- Osteoporosis (long-term use)

METABOLISM AND HALF-LIFE Metabolised by heparinase in liver and reticulo-endothelial cells. Metabolites are excreted in urine. $t_{\frac{1}{2}}$ is 2–4 h (prolonged in renal or hepatic failure).

MONITORING Monitoring is not routinely required. In LMWH toxicity there is no effective antidote.

DRUG INTERACTIONS
- Increased risk of bleeding with NSAIDs (including aspirin), warfarin, clopidogrel and dipyridamole
- Nitrate infusion reduces efficacy of LMWH

IMPORTANT POINTS
- Maximum plasma levels after subcutaneous injection are achieved more rapidly and bioavailability is improved
- Shorter half-life (approximately half that of unfractionated heparin)
- Predictable response reduces need for monitoring (monitored by measurement of anti-factor Xa activity instead of APTT in patients at increased risk of bleeding)
- As effective as unfractionated heparin in prevention and treatment of venous thrombo-embolism and associated with fewer bleeding complications
- Osteoporosis may occur in long-term use (usually >6 months)

Nitrates

EXAMPLES   Glyceryl trinitrate (GTN), isosorbide mononitrate (ISMN)

MECHANISM OF ACTION   Metabolised to nitric oxide that activates guanylyl cyclase, increasing production of cGMP in vascular tissues. This secondary messenger causes smooth muscle relaxation resulting in coronary artery dilatation (increasing oxygen supply to myocardium) and systemic venodilatation (reducing preload and thereby reducing oxygen demand).

INDICATIONS
- Prophylaxis and treatment of angina
- LVF

CAUTIONS AND CONTRA-INDICATIONS
- Hypersensitivity to nitrates
- Hypotension/hypovolaemia
- Cardiac outflow obstruction (aortic stenosis, cardiac tamponade, hypertrophic obstructive cardiomyopathy, constrictive pericarditis)
- Closed-angle glaucoma

SIDE-EFFECTS
- Postural hypotension
- Headache
- Tachycardia
- Dizziness

METABOLISM AND HALF-LIFE   Metabolised by the liver and other cells including red blood cells. $t_{1/2}$ is variable – for intravenous GTN $t_{1/2}$ is 4–6 min and for oral ISMN $t_{1/2}$ is ~6 h.

MONITORING   BP monitoring is required for intravenous infusion.

DRUG INTERACTIONS
- Reduce anticoagulant effect of low molecular weight heparin
- Risk of severe hypotension with phosphodiesterase type 5 inhibitors (e.g. sildenafil)

IMPORTANT POINTS
- Tolerance to nitrates may develop hence patients should have at least 8 h nitrate-free every 24 h (except when administered intravenously in the acute setting)

Potassium channel activators

EXAMPLES   Nicorandil

MECHANISM OF ACTION   Dual mechanism of action. Opens ATP-sensitive K^+ channels resulting in smooth muscle relaxation, thereby promoting arterial vasodilatation and reducing afterload. Nitric oxide moiety activates guanylyl cyclase to achieve venous relaxation and a reduction in preload. Direct effects on the coronary arteries are also seen.

INDICATIONS
- Prophylaxis and treatment of angina

CAUTIONS AND CONTRA-INDICATIONS
- Cardiogenic shock
- Hypotension
- LVF with poor filling pressures

SIDE-EFFECTS
- Headaches on initiation
- Nausea and vomiting
- Dizziness
- Flushing
- Weakness
- Oral ulceration
- Angioedema

METABOLISM AND HALF-LIFE $t_{1/2}$ is 40–80 min. Metabolised by the liver via nicotinamide pathway; <20% excreted in urine.

MONITORING   Monitor clinically for adverse effects.

DRUG INTERACTIONS
- Hypotensive effects significantly enhanced when taken with phosphodiesterase type 5 inhibitors (e.g. sildenafil)
- Hypotensive effects possibly enhanced with tricyclic antidepressants and alcohol

IMPORTANT POINTS
- Start at lower dose in patients susceptible to headaches
- Patients are advised not to drive or operate machinery until it is established that their performance is unaffected
- Titrate dose to symptomatic relief
- Used as an add-on therapy

Statins

EXAMPLES   Simvastatin, atorvastatin, pravastatin, rosuvastatin

MECHANISM OF ACTION   Inhibition of HMG CoA reductase, preventing hepatic conversion of mevalonic acid to cholesterol. Reduced cholesterol synthesis in the liver results in decreased plasma LDL.

INDICATIONS
- Prevention of cardiovascular events in patients with atherosclerotic disease or diabetes mellitus
- Primary hyperlipidaemia

CAUTIONS AND CONTRA-INDICATIONS
- Active liver disease (caution needed in patients with alcohol dependence)
- Pregnancy and breastfeeding

SIDE-EFFECTS
- Rhabdomyolysis (rare but may manifest as myalgia, myositis or myopathy)
- Altered liver function tests
- GI disturbance

METABOLISM AND HALF-LIFE   Metabolised by Cytochrome P450 (except pravastatin and rosuvastatin); clinical effects largely due to active metabolites. $t_{1/2}$ is variable – 2 h for simvastatin; 14 h for atorvastatin.

MONITORING   Patients should be warned about possible rhabdomyolysis; if suspected check creatine kinase level. LFTs should be checked 3 months following initiation.

DRUG INTERACTIONS
- Increased risk of myopathy with fibrates, amiodarone and calcium channel blockers
- Plasma concentration increased by grapefruit juice and macrolides
- Plasma concentration reduced by rifampicin

IMPORTANT POINTS
- Statins are more effective than any other lipid-lowering agents
- Greatest reduction of LDL is achieved with atorvastatin and rosuvastatin (60–65% reduction at maximum dose)

Thiazide diuretics

EXAMPLES   Bendroflumethiazide

MECHANISM OF ACTION   Inhibit Na^+/Cl^- symporter in the distal convoluted tubules thereby reducing Na^+ reabsorption and reducing water reabsorption.

INDICATIONS
- Hypertension
- Oedema in heart failure

CAUTIONS AND CONTRA-INDICATIONS
- Electrolyte disturbances (including refractory hypokalaemia, hyponatraemia, hypercalcaemia and symptomatic hyperuricaemia)
- Addison's disease
- Avoid in breastfeeding mothers due to suppression of lactation

SIDE-EFFECTS
- Postural hypotension
- Hyponatraemia
- Hypokalaemia
- Hyperuricaemia (e.g. gout)
- Hypercalcaemia
- Hyperglycaemia
- Male sexual dysfunction
- Suppression of lactation
- Raised LDL cholesterol

METABOLISM AND HALF-LIFE   Metabolised in the liver. $t_{1/2}$ is 3–4 h.

MONITORING   Monitor plasma electrolytes for adverse effects as above.

DRUG INTERACTIONS
- Enhanced hypotensive effect with other antihypertensives
- Increased risk of nephrotoxicity with NSAIDs
- Reduced hypoglycaemic effect of oral antidiabetic agents

IMPORTANT POINTS
- Thiazides are less effective than loop diuretics because 90% of Na^+ has been reabsorbed by the time the filtrate reaches the distal convoluted tubule
- Hypokalaemia results from increased activity of Na^+/K^+ ATPase in collecting ducts. This is caused by increased Na^+ in filtrate and an aldosterone-mediated effect (diuretic-induced hypovolaemia causes activation of the renin–angiotensin–aldosterone system)

Tranexamic acid

MECHANISM OF ACTION   Competitively inhibits the activation of plasminogen into plasmin, thereby reducing fibrin clot degradation. At high doses can directly inhibit plasmin activity.

INDICATIONS
- Menorrhagia
- Epistaxis
- Thrombolytic overdose
- Prevent excessive bleeding (dental extraction in haemophilia)

CAUTIONS AND CONTRA-INDICATIONS
- Thromboembolic disease

SIDE-EFFECTS
- GI disturbance
- Disturbance in colour vision

METABOLISM AND HALF-LIFE   Plasma $t_{1/2}$ is between 2–3 h.

MONITORING   No specific drug monitoring required. Eye tests for long-term treatment.

DRUG INTERACTIONS
- Counters the effects of fibrinolytic agents (e.g. streptokinase, alteplase)

IMPORTANT POINTS
- Treatment should be initiated during menstruation when managing menorrhagia

Vasoconstrictor sympathomimetics

EXAMPLES   Noradrenaline, ephedrine, phenylephrine

MECHANISM OF ACTION   Stimulation of peripheral α-adrenoceptors within vasculature, leading to vasoconstriction and increased systolic and diastolic blood pressure

INDICATIONS
- Acute hypotension
- Cardiac arrest

CAUTIONS AND CONTRA-INDICATIONS
- Hypertension

SIDE-EFFECTS
- Hypertension
- Headache
- Arrhythmias
- Bradycardia/tachycardia

METABOLISM AND HALF-LIFE   Metabolised in the liver and other tissues by MAO and COMT.

MONITORING   Continuous cardiac monitoring in a high-dependency area is required. Monitoring of oxygen saturation, urine output and renal function is also necessary.

DRUG INTERACTIONS
- Severe, prolonged hypertension when given in combination with MAOIs

IMPORTANT POINTS
- Ephedrine can be used to treat hypotension resulting from spinal/epidural anaesthesia
- See Inotropic sympathomimetics, p.26

Warfarin

MECHANISM OF ACTION Coumarin anticoagulant; inhibits hepatic synthesis of vitamin K-dependent clotting factors (II, VII, IX, X) and co-factors (proteins C and S). Thus the predominant action of warfarin is on the extrinsic pathway of the clotting cascade.

INDICATIONS
- DVT
- PE
- Prophylaxis of VTE in AF, rheumatic heart disease and in patients with prosthetic heart valves

CAUTIONS AND CONTRA-INDICATIONS
- Peptic ulceration
- Severe hypertension
- Pregnancy (due to teratogenicity)
- Caution if recent surgery

SIDE-EFFECTS
- Haemorrhage
- Hypersensitivity/rash
- Hepatic dysfunction
- Skin necrosis (due to thrombosis in microvasculature of subcutaneous fat)

METABOLISM AND HALF-LIFE $t_{1/2}$ is ~37 h; metabolised by liver.

MONITORING Monitor INR (initially daily and then at progressively lengthening intervals when steady INR is achieved).

DRUG INTERACTIONS (this list is not exhaustive)
- Anticoagulant effect of warfarin is increased by:
  - Antibiotics (due to reduced vitamin K synthesis by gut flora)
  - Amiodarone and diuretics (displace warfarin from plasma proteins)
  - Cimetidine, fluconazole, alcohol (reduce metabolism of warfarin)
  - Aspirin, clopidogrel, NSAIDs (due to impaired platelet function)
  - Also by advanced age, biliary disease, CCF, hyperthyroidism, cranberry juice and intermittent alcohol binges
- Anticoagulant effect of warfarin is reduced by:
  - Antiepileptic agents, rifampicin, alcoholism (due to induction of hepatic enzymes)
  - Oestrogens and OCP (increase concentration of vitamin K-dependent clotting factors)
  - Also by hypothyroidism and nephritic syndrome

IMPORTANT POINTS
- Effects on proteins C and S precede anticoagulant effect thereby transiently increasing risk of thrombosis; anticoagulation with heparin should therefore be used concomitantly for at least 5 days and until INR is within target range for treatment of a thrombotic event
- Target INR depends on indication (e.g. 2.0–3.0 for VTE and AF; 3.0–4.5 for prosthetic heart valves; 4.0–5.0 for high-risk heart valves)
- Vitamin K may be used to reverse anticoagulation with warfarin; use should be limited to major bleeding or high INR in a patient with other risk factors for bleeding
- Prothrombin complex concentrate may also be used to reverse effects of warfarin in severe bleeding

β_2 adrenoceptor agonists

EXAMPLES   Short-acting – salbutamol, terbutaline; long-acting – salmeterol, formoterol.

MECHANISM OF ACTION   Selective β_2 adrenoceptor agonists in smooth muscle of upper airways that increase intracellular cAMP. This leads to smooth muscle relaxation and bronchodilation.

INDICATIONS
- Acute asthma (short-acting)
- Chronic asthma/COPD (long-acting)
- Premature labour

CAUTIONS AND CONTRA-INDICATIONS
- Hypersensitivity

SIDE-EFFECTS
- Fine tremor
- Hypokalaemia (if high doses given)
- Tachycardia
- Headache

METABOLISM AND HALF-LIFE   The effects of long-acting drugs last $\sim$12 h. Proportion reaching GI tract is metabolised by the liver. $t_{1/2}$ varies; salbutamol 3–7 h; terbutaline 16–20 h.

MONITORING   Monitor K^+ levels if high doses of salbutamol given (especially in acute asthma).

DRUG INTERACTIONS
- Should not be given with non-selective β_2 blockers, due to opposing actions
- In management of acute asthma, hypokalaemia may be potentiated by hypoxia and the use of theophylline, steroids and diuretics

IMPORTANT POINTS
- Salbutamol can be administered by inhaler, nebuliser or IV in the management of acute asthma
- Salbutamol can be used in the immediate management of hyperkalaemia (increases uptake of K^+ into cells)
- BTS guidelines recommend a stepwise approach to the management of chronic asthma. First-line therapy involves the use of short-acting β_2 agonists; if symptoms are uncontrolled this is supplemented with inhaled corticosteroids and then long-acting β_2 agonists
- β_2 agonists salbutamol and terbutaline can be used to delay uncomplicated premature labour (24–33 weeks gestation) by at least 48 h, by inhibition of uterine contractions

Histamine type 1 receptor antagonists

EXAMPLES Cetirizine, chlorphenamine, desloratadine, fexofenadine

MECHANISM OF ACTION Competitive inhibition at H_1 receptors, blocking the acute inflammatory effects of histamine (i.e. vasodilatation, increased vascular permeability and pain). Some also have antimuscarinic effects resulting in drowsiness and contributing to an anti-emetic effect (see Antihistamine anti-emetics, p.44).

INDICATIONS
- Symptomatic relief of allergy (e.g. seasonal allergic rhinitis)
- Pruritus
- Urticaria
- Emergency treatment of anaphylaxis and angioedema (chlorphenamine)

CAUTIONS AND CONTRA-INDICATIONS
- Prostatic hypertrophy
- Urinary retention
- Susceptibility to closed-angle glaucoma

SIDE-EFFECTS
- Sedation (particularly chlorphenamine and hydroxyzine)
- Rarely paradoxical excitation in children and elderly
- Antimuscarinic effects (urinary retention, dry mouth, blurred vision and GI disturbance)

METABOLISM AND HALF-LIFE Highly variable $t_{1/2}$ from 12–43 h.

MONITORING No specific drug monitoring required.

DRUG INTERACTIONS
- Concurrent use of hypnotics, anxiolytics or alcohol may exacerbate drowsiness
- Increased antimuscarinic effects when given with MAOIs or TCAs

IMPORTANT POINTS
- Antihistamines are broadly divided into sedating (e.g. chlorphenamine) and non-sedating agents (e.g. cetirizine, desloratadine, fexofenadine)
- Drowsiness frequently diminishes after the first few days of treatment but patients should be advised of this adverse effect as it may affect their ability to perform tasks, including driving

Inhaled antimuscarinics

EXAMPLES   Ipratropium bromide, tiotropium

MECHANISM OF ACTION   Competitive antagonists of acetylcholine in bronchial smooth muscle. Inhaled antimuscarinics bind to and block muscarinic (M_3) receptors, thereby preventing smooth muscle contraction and consequent airway constriction.

INDICATIONS
- Asthma (ipratropium bromide only)
- COPD

CAUTIONS AND CONTRA-INDICATIONS
- Caution in patients susceptible to closed-angle glaucoma

SIDE-EFFECTS
- Dry mouth
- Nausea
- Headache
- Other systemic side-effects may occur but are rare (see Antimuscarinics, p.14)

METABOLISM AND HALF-LIFE   Depending on formulation, device and adequacy of administration technique 10–30% of dose reaches the airways. $t_{1/2}$ for ipratropium bromide is ~1.6 h and for tiotropium is 5–6 days; both are predominantly excreted in urine.

MONITORING   No specific drug monitoring required.

DRUG INTERACTIONS
- Increased risk of adverse effects if co-administered with other anticholinergic agents

IMPORTANT POINTS
- Ipratropium bromide is used predominantly in COPD but can be used in a nebulised form with salbutamol for acute asthma not responsive to standard therapy
- The maximal effect of ipratropium bromide is achieved 30–60 min after administration and the duration of action is 3–6 h
- Tiotropium is a long-acting agent that is not suitable for treatment of acute bronchospasm

Leukotriene receptor antagonists

EXAMPLES   Montelukast, zafirlukast

MECHANISM OF ACTION   Block the action of cysteinyl leukotrienes (pro-inflammatory eicosanoids released from mast cells and eosinophils) in the smooth muscle of the airways, thereby inhibiting the inflammation responsible for symptomatic asthma and rhinitis.

INDICATIONS
- Prophylaxis of asthma
- Seasonal allergic rhinitis

CAUTIONS AND CONTRA-INDICATIONS
- Hypersensitivity
- Hepatic impairment (zafirlukast)

SIDE-EFFECTS
- Abdominal pain
- GI disturbance
- Headache

METABOLISM AND HALF-LIFE   Metabolised extensively by the liver and excreted via the biliary route. $t_{1/2}$ varies: zafirlukast 10 h; montelukast 3–7 h.

MONITORING   No specific drug monitoring required.

DRUG INTERACTIONS
- Caution in patients taking liver enzyme inducing drugs: phenytoin and rifampicin
- Plasma levels reduced co-administration with phenobarbital

IMPORTANT POINTS
- BTS guidelines recommend a stepwise approach to the management of chronic asthma. Leukotriene receptor antagonists can be used as single therapy or with an inhaled steroid (their effects are additive)
- Leukotriene receptor antagonists may be of benefit in exercise-induced asthma
- Montelukast is given as a once daily oral preparation whilst zafirlukast is given as a twice daily dose

Oxygen

MECHANISM OF ACTION   Oxygen is the terminal electron acceptor in the oxidative phosphorylation pathway and is thus an essential component of the electron transport chains that produce ATP. In the absence of oxygen, pyruvate produced from glycolysis is converted into lactate.

INDICATIONS
- Hypoxaemia (oxygen should be titrated to achieve a target saturation of 94–98% for most acutely ill patients and 88–92% for those at risk of hypercapnic respiratory failure pending blood gas results).

CAUTIONS AND CONTRA-INDICATIONS
- Caution in patients at risk of hypercapnic respiratory failure (although oxygen should not be withheld from acutely hypoxaemic patients).

SIDE-EFFECTS
- Respiratory depression in patients reliant upon hypoxic drive
- Coronary and cerebral vasoconstriction
- Oxygen toxicity from free radicals
- Rebound hypoxaemia following sudden cessation of oxygen therapy

MONITORING   Pulse oximetry monitoring is required supplemented by blood gas analysis. Oxygen flow rates and delivery system should be adjusted to maintain oxygen saturation within target range.

DRUG INTERACTIONS
- Potentiates lung injury due to paraquat poisoning, ingestion of acids or damage due to bleomycin therapy

IMPORTANT POINTS
- Oxygen should be prescribed in a patient's drug chart
- Low-flow systems (dependent on flow rate and respiratory pattern)
  - Nasal prongs: FiO_2 up to 40%
  - Face mask: FiO_2 up to 60%
  - Face mask with reservoir bag: FiO_2 up to 100%
- High-flow systems (fixed-flow rate and independent of respiratory pattern)
  - Venturi mask: FiO_2 24–60%

Theophylline

MECHANISM OF ACTION   A methylxanthine that inhibits phosphodiesterase isoenzymes resulting in increased cAMP levels and smooth muscle relaxation, hence has a bronchodilatory effect on the airways. Theophylline also acts as a respiratory stimulant through the CNS.

INDICATIONS
- Acute severe asthma
- Chronic asthma
- Moderate to severe COPD

CAUTIONS AND CONTRA-INDICATIONS
- Porphyria
- Concomitant use of ephedrine in children
- Caution should be exercised in cardiac or liver failure and poorly controlled epilepsy (consider dose reduction)

SIDE-EFFECTS
- Hypokalaemia
- Tachycardia, palpitations and arrhythmias
- Headache and insomnia
- GI disturbances (especially nausea)
- Convulsions, especially if given rapidly by IV injection

METABOLISM AND HALF-LIFE   Extensively metabolised by the liver to metabolites that are excreted via the kidneys. $t_{1/2}$ is between 3–9 h.

MONITORING   Levels are measured 4–6 hours after a dose and should be checked within 5 days after starting treatment. Narrow therapeutic index. Monitor K^+ levels. Cardiac monitoring recommended for IV doses.

DRUG INTERACTIONS
- Metabolised extensively via Cytochrome P450 and thus multiple drug interactions
- Theophylline levels increased with CCBs, cimetidine, quinolones, macrolides and some antifungals (e.g. ketoconazole and fluconazole)
- Theophylline levels are decreased in smokers, chronic alcohol intake and by drugs that induce liver metabolism, such as antiepileptics and rifampicin

IMPORTANT POINTS
- Toxicity may be delayed with modified release preparations. Clinical features include vomiting and agitation. Haematemesis, cardiac arrhythmias and convulsions are potentially life-threatening
- In overdose, patients need continuous cardiac monitoring and regular blood monitoring (hypokalaemia is potentiated by β_2 agonists and hyperglycaemia)
- Aminophylline is a combination of theophylline and ethylenediamine; the latter confers water soluble properties and hence aminophylline is used as an IV preparation

5-HT₁ agonists (triptans)

EXAMPLES   Sumatriptan, zolmitriptan

MECHANISM OF ACTION   Selective activation of 5-HT$_1$ receptors that are predominantly located in cranial blood vessel walls. 5-HT$_1$ receptors mediate vasoconstriction thereby relieving symptoms that are believed to result from the dilatation of intra- and extracranial vessels.

INDICATIONS
• Treatment of acute migraine
• Cluster headache

CAUTIONS AND CONTRA-INDICATIONS
• Ischaemic heart disease or coronary vasospasm
• Peripheral vascular disease
• Previous stroke or TIA
• Severe hypertension

SIDE-EFFECTS
• Dizziness
• Paraesthesia
• Tinnitus
• Transient rise in blood pressure
• Tachycardia and palpitations
• Very rarely, MI

METABOLISM AND HALF-LIFE   Eliminated via metabolism by MAO-A. $t_{1/2}$ is 2–6 h.

MONITORING   No specific drug monitoring required.

DRUG INTERACTIONS
• Increased risk of CNS toxicity with SSRIs and MAOIs
• Plasma concentration of 5-HT$_1$ agonists may be increased by macrolides and β blockers

IMPORTANT POINTS
• 5-HT$_1$ agonists are the preferred treatment for patients with migraines that do not respond to simple analgesia
• 5-HT$_1$ agonists should be used in the established headache phase of an attack; they are not suitable for migraine prophylaxis
• Newer formulations include SC preparations, IN preparations and wafers for faster administration

5-HT$_3$ antagonists

EXAMPLES   Ondansetron, granisetron

MECHANISM OF ACTION   Selective 5-HT$_3$ receptor antagonists that act peripherally on vagal nerve endings of the GI tract and centrally in the CTZ. 5-HT$_3$ receptors in the CTZ in the area postrema of the medulla contribute to the perception of nausea and the control of vomiting.

INDICATIONS
- PONV
- Nausea and vomiting associated with cytotoxic drugs (chemotherapy) and radiotherapy

CAUTIONS AND CONTRA-INDICATIONS
- Prolonged QT interval and cardiac conduction defects
- Hypersensitivity

SIDE-EFFECTS
- GI disturbance (especially constipation due to increased large bowel transit time)
- Headache
- Flushing

METABOLISM AND HALF-LIFE   Metabolised predominantly in the liver. $t_{1/2}$ for ondansetron and granisetron is ~5 h.

MONITORING   No specific drug monitoring required.

DRUG INTERACTIONS
- Effects reduced by drugs that induce liver enzymes (phenytoin, carbamazepine, rifampicin)
- Increased risk of torsades de pointes with other drugs that prolong the QT interval

IMPORTANT POINTS
- Establish a cause for emesis prior to prescribing an anti-emetic
- Very effective anti-emetic agents, particularly for PONV
- Careful monitoring of symptoms if these drugs are used in patients with subacute bowel obstruction due to effects on large bowel motility

Antihistamine anti-emetics

EXAMPLES   Cyclizine, promethazine

MECHANISM OF ACTION H_1 receptor antagonists directly inhibit the CTZ in the medulla. They possess anticholinergic and anti-emetic properties. Cyclizine also increases lower oesophageal sphincter tone and reduces the sensitivity of the labyrinthine apparatus.

INDICATIONS
- Nausea and vomiting
- Hyperemesis in pregnancy (promethazine is first line)
- Vomiting in labyrinthine disorders
- Nausea associated with motion sickness

CAUTIONS AND CONTRA-INDICATIONS
- Severe prostatic hypertrophy
- Caution in patients at risk of closed-angle glaucoma

SIDE-EFFECTS
- Drowsiness
- Headache
- Tachycardia (cyclizine)
- Psychomotor impairment
- Antimuscarinic effects

METABOLISM AND HALF-LIFE   Metabolised by the liver to an inactive metabolite. $t_{1/2}$ for cyclizine is $\sim$20 h.

MONITORING   No specific drug monitoring required.

DRUG INTERACTIONS
- Increased sedative effect with opiates

IMPORTANT POINTS
- Establish a cause for emesis prior to prescribing an anti-emetic
- Sedative effects of antihistamines are likely to be potentiated in liver disease
- Cyclizine and promethazine are safe to prescribe in pregnancy

Antipsychotics – atypical

EXAMPLES Clozapine, olanzapine, quetiapine, risperidone, amisulpride

MECHANISM OF ACTION Not a homogenous pharmacological class. Atypical antipsychotics act predominantly via dopamine (D_1 to D_4) and 5-HT receptors (See also Phenothiazine anti-emetics, p.60)

INDICATIONS
- Schizophrenia and other psychoses
- Mania
- Sedation
- Anxiety and psychomotor agitation

CAUTIONS AND CONTRA-INDICATIONS
- CNS depression and coma
- Severe cardiovascular disease
- Caution in patients with hepatic impairment
- Caution in epilepsy
- Caution in elderly patients and patients with risk factors for cerebrovascular disease (increased risk of stroke in older patients with dementia with olanzapine and risperidone)

SIDE-EFFECTS
- Sedation or agitation
- Postural hypotension
- Antimuscarinic effects
- Weight gain
- Neutropenia and agranulocytosis (clozapine only)
- Myocarditis and cardiomyopathy (clozapine only)
- Hyperglycaemia (particularly clozapine and olanzapine)
- Rarely, neuroleptic malignant syndrome

METABOLISM AND HALF-LIFE Variable $t_{1/2}$; most are largely metabolised by the liver prior to excretion.

MONITORING Check FBC prior to starting clozapine and initially monitor counts weekly. Cardiovascular assessment prior to starting clozapine.

DRUG INTERACTIONS
- Antagonism of sympathomimetics, anticholinergics and antiepileptic drugs may occur (the latter may lower seizure threshold)
- Enhanced hypotensive effect with antihypertensive agents
- Increased risk of cardiac arrhythmias (including torsades de pointes) with other drugs that prolong the QT interval

IMPORTANT POINTS
- NICE guidance recommends that atypical antipsychotics should be considered as first-line agents for newly diagnosed schizophrenia but that, where possible, the choice of agent should be discussed with the patient prior to initiation
- Atypical antipsychotics are more effective in the treatment of negative symptoms of schizophrenia
- Withdrawal of antipsychotics after long-term therapy should be gradual to avoid the risk of acute withdrawal or rebound psychosis
- If a treatment is effective but compliance is poor, depot preparations may be considered

Antipsychotics – typical

EXAMPLES   Haloperidol, chlorpromazine, prochlorperazine, flupentixol

MECHANISM OF ACTION   Not a homogenous pharmacological class. Mixed antagonists at muscarinic, histaminergic, dopaminergic, serotonergic and adrenergic receptors. Typical antipsychotics exert their predominant neuroleptic effect through blockade of dopamine D_2 receptors.

INDICATIONS
- Schizophrenia and other psychoses
- Mania
- Sedation
- Anxiety and psychomotor agitation
- Nausea and vomiting

CAUTIONS AND CONTRA-INDICATIONS
- CNS depression and coma
- Severe cardiovascular disease
- Caution in patients with hepatic impairment
- Caution in epilepsy

SIDE-EFFECTS
- Sedation or agitation
- Extra-pyramidal symptoms
- Postural hypotension
- Cardiac arrhythmias (prolongation of QT interval)
- Antimuscarinic effects
- Hyperprolactinaemia
- Rarely, neuroleptic malignant syndrome

METABOLISM AND HALF-LIFE   Variable $t_{1/2}$; most are largely metabolised by the liver prior to excretion.

MONITORING   ECG before initiating treatment and then annually with some typical antipsychotics.

DRUG INTERACTIONS
- Phenothiazines (e.g. chlorpromazine, prochlorperazine) may enhance the CNS depressant effect of opioids, anxiolytics, sedatives, hypnotics and alcohol
- Antagonism of sympathomimetics, anticholinergics and antiepileptic drugs may occur (the latter may lower seizure threshold)
- Enhanced hypotensive effect with antihypertensive agents
- Increased risk of cardiac arrhythmias (including torsades de pointes) with other drugs that prolong the QT interval

IMPORTANT POINTS
- Withdrawal of antipsychotics after long-term therapy should be gradual to avoid the risk of acute withdrawal or rebound psychosis
- If a treatment is effective but compliance is poor, depot preparations may be considered

Benzodiazepines

EXAMPLES   Diazepam, lorazepam, chlordiazepoxide, midazolam, temazepam

MECHANISM OF ACTION   Bind to benzodiazepine receptors that are coupled to GABA receptors. This increases the affinity of GABA to its receptor and opens Cl^- channels resulting in hyperpolarisation of the cell membrane, thereby preventing further excitation.

INDICATIONS
- Short-term use in anxiety or insomnia
- Acute alcohol withdrawal
- Sedation
- Status epilepticus
- Muscle spasm

CAUTIONS AND CONTRA-INDICATIONS
- Respiratory depression
- Neuromuscular disease affecting muscles of respiration
- Acute pulmonary insufficiency
- Should not be used as monotherapy to treat depression (with or without anxiety)

SIDE-EFFECTS
- Drowsiness and lightheadedness
- Dependence
- Confusion
- Amnesia

METABOLISM AND HALF-LIFE   Extensive hepatic metabolism. $t_{1/2}$ is variable; midazolam is short-acting ($t_{1/2}$ 1–8 h); temazepam is intermediate-acting ($t_{1/2}$ 8–40 h) and diazepam and chlordiazepoxide are long-acting ($t_{1/2}$ 40–200 h).

MONITORING   Monitor respiratory effort and effect (respiratory rate and oxygen saturations).

DRUG INTERACTIONS
- Should not be taken with alcohol due to increased sedative effect

IMPORTANT POINTS
- Effect of excessive benzodiazepine use can be reversed by flumazenil. This is administered via IV route
- Chlordiazepoxide can be used to lessen the symptoms of alcohol withdrawal. Chlordiazepoxide is given for a limited time (3–10 days) in reducing doses but should not be given if a patient is likely to continue drinking alcohol

Carbamazepine

MECHANISM OF ACTION   Use-dependent blockade of voltage-gated Na^+ channels responsible for propagation of the action potential. Thus carbamazepine preferentially blocks the excitation of neurones that are firing repeatedly.

INDICATIONS
- Epilepsy
- Prophylaxis of bipolar disorder
- Trigeminal neuralgia

CAUTIONS AND CONTRA-INDICATIONS
- AV conduction abnormalities (if not paced)
- History of bone marrow suppression
- Acute porphyria

SIDE-EFFECTS
- Nausea and vomiting
- Drowsiness
- Generalised erythematous rash
- Cardiac conduction disturbances
- Leucopenia

METABOLISM AND HALF-LIFE   Metabolised by the liver by Cytochrome P450 3A4. $t_{1/2}$ is 16–36 h.

MONITORING   No specific drug monitoring required.

DRUG INTERACTIONS
- Plasma levels can be enhanced by drugs inhibiting Cytochrome P450, including isoniazid, verapamil and diltiazem
- Plasma levels can be reduced by drugs that potentiate Cytochrome P450, including phenytoin, phenobarbitone and theophylline
- Reduces anticoagulant effect of warfarin
- Anticonvulsant effect antagonised by antipsychotics

IMPORTANT POINTS
- Treatment should be started at a low dose with small incremental increases every 2 weeks
- Carbamazepine can be used in the prophylaxis of bipolar disorder if symptoms are not responding to lithium

Dopamine antagonist anti-emetics

EXAMPLES Domperidone, metoclopramide

MECHANISM OF ACTION The anti-emetic effect is due to a combination of prokinetic activity, up-regulation of the parasympathetic nervous system and antagonism of dopamine D_2 receptors in the CTZ.

INDICATIONS
• Nausea and vomiting

CAUTIONS AND CONTRA-INDICATIONS
• Phaeochromocytoma
• Prolactin-releasing pituitary tumour
• GI obstruction
• Perforation

SIDE-EFFECTS
• Extra-pyramidal symptoms
• Hyperprolactinaemia
• Neuroleptic malignant syndrome
• Rashes
• Tardive dyskinesia
• Confusion
• Drowsiness

METABOLISM AND HALF-LIFE Extensive hepatic metabolism by hydroxylation. Domperidone has $t_{1/2}$ of 7–9 h.

MONITORING No specific drug monitoring required.

DRUG INTERACTIONS
• Metoclopramide increases plasma levels of ciclosporin and NSAIDs
• Ketoconazole increases risk of arrhythmias when given with domperidone

IMPORTANT POINTS
• Always establish a cause for vomiting prior to prescribing anti-emetics
• Dopamine antagonists can cause severe extra-pyramidal side-effects when given to young adults and elderly patients
• Dopamine antagonists are particularly useful in vomiting secondary to chemotherapy and radiotherapy

Drugs for dementia

MECHANISM OF ACTION

Donepezil, galantamine and rivastigmine – inhibition of acetylcholinesterase thereby preventing the breakdown of ACh; the cholinergic hypothesis suggests that reduced ACh synthesis is a key aetiological factor in Alzheimer's disease. Galantamine also acts as a partial agonist at nicotinic receptors.

Memantine – NMDA receptor antagonist that blocks the effects of pathologically elevated levels of glutamate that may contribute to neuronal dysfunction in Alzheimer's disease.

INDICATIONS

- Mild to moderate dementia in Alzheimer's disease
- Mild to moderate dementia in Parkinson's disease (rivastigmine only)

CAUTIONS AND CONTRA-INDICATIONS

- Caution in cardiac disease
- Caution in asthma/COPD
- Caution in patients susceptible to peptic ulcers
- Caution in renal impairment

SIDE-EFFECTS

- GI disturbance
- Gastric or duodenal ulcers
- Drowsiness and confusion
- Rarely, arrhythmias and SA node/AV node block

METABOLISM AND HALF-LIFE Variable – e.g. $t_{1/2}$ ~70 h for donepezil; $t_{1/2}$ ~1 h for rivastigmine.

MONITORING Monitor MMSE score every 6 months – treatment should only be continued while score remains at or above 10 (out of 30).

DRUG INTERACTIONS

- Increased risk of arrhythmias with agents that reduce heart rate (e.g. β blockers, digoxin, amiodarone)
- Effects antagonised by antimuscarinics

IMPORTANT POINTS

- Exclude reversible causes of cognitive impairment prior to initiating treatment (e.g. hypothyroidism)
- Drugs for dementia should only be started by specialists
- NICE guidance (2007) recommends the use of acetylcholinesterase inhibitors in patients with a MMSE score between 10 and 20 points. NICE does not recommend memantine for routine use
- The clinical benefits of acetylcholinesterase inhibitors are modest with only about a 10% improvement in short-term memory, language and praxis abilities at best

Gabapentin and pregabalin

MECHANISM OF ACTION   Exact mechanism is unclear. Gabapentin and pregabalin are analogues of GABA. Their clinical benefits are not mediated by the action on GABA receptors within the CNS but through binding to a subunit on T-type Ca^{2+} channels and selectively inhibiting the release of various neurotransmitters. Pregabalin is a higher potency analogue of gabapentin in chronic pain control.

INDICATIONS
- Partial seizures with or without secondary generalisation (as monotherapy or adjunct)
- Neuropathic pain

CAUTIONS AND CONTRA-INDICATIONS
- Hypersensitivity

SIDE-EFFECTS
- GI disturbance
- Weight gain
- Hypertension
- Dizziness and drowsiness
- Leucopenia
- Visual disturbances (e.g. diplopia)

METABOLISM AND HALF-LIFE   Gabapentin is eliminated unchanged solely by renal excretion; $t_{1/2}$ is 5–7 h. Pregabalin has a similar profile.

MONITORING   No specific drug monitoring required.

DRUG INTERACTIONS
- Increased risk of CNS depression with opiates
- Antacids containing aluminium and magnesium can reduce gabapentin bioavailability

IMPORTANT POINTS
- Abrupt withdrawal can cause anxiety, insomnia, pain and increases risk of seizures in epileptics
- Lower doses should be considered in the elderly and patients with renal impairment
- Gabapentin should be started at a low dose and gradually increased in increments over 2–3 days. Sedation, confusion and ataxia have been reported with rapid titration

Levodopa (L-dopa)

MECHANISM OF ACTION   Metabolic precursor of dopamine. Acts on all dopamine receptors in dopamine-depleted regions within the striatum, pallidum and substantia nigra of the basal ganglia.

INDICATIONS
- Parkinson's disease and parkinsonism

CAUTIONS AND CONTRA-INDICATIONS
- Hypersensitivity
- Closed-angle glaucoma
- Severe neuropsychosis
- Severe heart failure and cardiac arrhythmias

SIDE-EFFECTS
- GI disturbance
- Dry mouth
- Postural hypotension
- Drowsiness and sudden onset of sleeping
- Dystonia, dyskinesia and chorea
- Neuropsychiatric symptoms: hallucinations, confusion, abnormal dreams, insomnia

METABOLISM AND HALF-LIFE $t_{1/2}$ is ~90 min but prolonged in the elderly. Metabolism is by decarboxylation to form dopamine and in turn is converted to inactive metabolites (and to a lesser extent to noradrenaline).

MONITORING   Monitor BP prior to and during treatment due to the risk of postural hypotension.

DRUG INTERACTIONS
- Increased risk of postural hypotension with antihypertensives
- Risk of hypertensive crisis with MAOIs

IMPORTANT POINTS
- L-dopa is given with a peripheral decarboxylase inhibitor to prevent the breakdown of L-dopa prior to reaching its target sites within the CNS and to reduce side-effects of peripheral dopamine action (e.g. nausea)
- 'On–off effect': sudden loss of antiparkinsonian effect of L-dopa that leads to hypokinesia and rigidity. Reduced efficacy of L-dopa may last for several hours. Counter-measures include reducing drug dose but increasing frequency
- 'End-of-dose' deterioration: duration of benefits after each dose becomes shortened. Modified-release preparations may be helpful
- Patients should be counselled on risk of sedation and sudden onset of sleep

Lithium

MECHANISM OF ACTION The precise mechanism as a mood stabiliser is unclear. It has been postulated that lithium interferes with the phosphatidyl-inositol pathway and negatively affects hormone-induced cAMP production.

INDICATIONS
- Treatment and prophylaxis of mania
- Prophylaxis of bipolar disorder

CAUTIONS AND CONTRA-INDICATIONS
- Renal disease
- Untreated hypothyroidism
- Severe cardiac disease
- Addison's disease
- Breastfeeding

SIDE-EFFECTS
- GI disturbance
- Fine tremor (common)
- Hyperparathyroidism and hypercalcaemia
- Weight gain and oedema
- Polyuria (inhibits antidiuretic hormone)
- Hypothyroidism

METABOLISM AND HALF-LIFE Excreted by the kidney – 50% of oral dose is usually excreted within 12 h. $t_{1/2}$ of lithium varies considerably but generally is considered to be about 12–24 h.

MONITORING Check U&Es, LFTs and TFTs prior to initiating treatment. Measure serum lithium concentration every 3 months (narrow therapeutic index). Monitor U&Es and TFTs every 6–12 months on stabilised regimens.

DRUG INTERACTIONS
- Increased risk of lithium toxicity with diuretics, ACEIs and ARBs due to reduced renal excretion
- NSAIDs reduce lithium excretion (reduce afferent arteriolar vasoconstriction)
- Increased risk of ventricular arrhythmias with amiodarone

IMPORTANT POINTS
- Preparations have different bioavailability
- Beneficial effects take 3–4 weeks to be seen
- Dehydration, reduced renal perfusion and infections predispose to lithium toxicity
- In overdose, toxic effects may clinically manifest with coarse tremor, worsening GI symptoms, blurred vision, drowsiness, ataxia and dysarthria and subsequently convulsions, psychosis and renal failure

Monoamine oxidase inhibitors (MAOIs)

EXAMPLES Phenelzine, moclobemide, selegiline

MECHANISM OF ACTION Inhibit MAO that degrades monoaminergic neurotransmitters in the synaptic cleft. There are two main subtypes of MAO – MAO-A breaks down adrenaline, noradrenaline, serotonin and melatonin; MAO-B breaks down phenethylamine; both subtypes degrade dopamine. Some agents (e.g. phenelzine) are non-subtype specific whereas others are specific (e.g. moclobemide is selective for MAO-A, selegiline is selective for MAO-B).

INDICATIONS
- Resistant depression particularly if atypical or hysterical features
- Parkinson's disease especially if problematic end-of-dose deterioration (MAO-B inhibitors only)

CAUTIONS AND CONTRA-INDICATIONS
- Hepatic dysfunction
- Phaeochromocytoma (due to risk of hypertensive crisis)
- Cerebrovascular disease

SIDE-EFFECTS
- Postural hypotension
- GI disturbance
- Headache and dizziness
- Rarely, hepatocellular necrosis
- Monoaminergic crisis (see below)

METABOLISM AND HALF-LIFE Eliminated entirely by metabolism, predominantly in liver. $t_{1/2}$ is 1–4 h.

MONITORING Monitor clinically for adverse effects.

DRUG INTERACTIONS
- Accumulation of amine neurotransmitters may result in a hypertensive crisis, hyperpyrexia and psychosis. It occurs with numerous agents including:
  o Sympathomimetics (e.g. in cough or decongestant medications)
  o SSRIs and TCAs
  o Levodopa
  o Opioid analgesics (especially pethidine)
  o Tyramine-containing foods (e.g. mature cheese, broad beans, beer, Marmite®)

IMPORTANT POINTS
- MAOIs are best avoided due to their potentially severe side-effects; adverse effects are less with selective agents particularly MAO-B inhibitors
- MAOIs should be withdrawn slowly due to physiological dependence and a consequent withdrawal syndrome
- Due to irreversible MAO inhibition other antidepressants should not be started for at least 2 weeks after stopping MAOIs
- Moclobemide is a reversible MAO-A inhibitor and therefore less problematic but it is reserved as second-line treatment

Non-steroidal anti-inflammatory drugs (NSAIDs)

EXAMPLES   Ibuprofen, diclofenac, naproxen, indometacin

MECHANISM OF ACTION   Non-selective inhibition of COX enzymes, COX-1 and COX-2. Inhibiting the production of prostaglandins and thromboxanes from arachidonic acid dampens the hyperalgesic and vasodilatory effects in acute inflammation. NSAIDs interrupt the synthesis of interleukin-1-mediated prostaglandin E in the hypothalamus resulting in an antipyretic effect. The analgesic and anti-inflammatory effects are attributed to a reduction in prostaglandins that normally sensitise nerve endings to these pain mediators.

INDICATIONS
- Mild to moderate pain
- Inflammatory musculoskeletal disorders
- Acute gout (excluding aspirin)
- Fever

CAUTIONS AND CONTRA-INDICATIONS
- History of active peptic ulcers
- Hypersensitivity

SIDE-EFFECTS
- GI disturbance
- Hypersensitivity reactions such as rashes
- Renal impairment
- Fluid retention
- Headaches and dizziness
- Bronchospasm

METABOLISM AND HALF-LIFE   Variable; e.g. $t_{1/2}$ for ibuprofen is $\sim$2 h. NSAIDs are excreted via the kidneys.

MONITORING   No specific drug monitoring required, unless patients have renal impairment.

DRUG INTERACTIONS
- Increased risk of nephrotoxicity when given with other potentially nephrotoxic drugs
- NSAIDs reduce lithium excretion
- NSAIDs can enhance the effects of warfarin

IMPORTANT POINTS
- COX-2 selective inhibitors (e.g. celecoxib, etoricoxib) are associated with an increased risk of thrombotic events (e.g. MI and stroke) but lower risk of GI side-effects than non-selective NSAIDs
- Acute renal failure may be provoked by NSAIDs, particularly in elderly and hypovalaemic patients. NSAIDs reduce glomerular filtration pressure by reducing prostaglandin production and resulting in constriction of the renal afferent arterioles
- The risk of adverse effects with NSAIDs is generally proportional to their potency, e.g. 'mild' ibuprofen compared with more 'potent' indometacin. Therefore, it is preferable to start with a low dose of a less potent drug

Opioid analgesia

EXAMPLES   Weak opioids – codeine, tramadol; strong opioids – fentanyl, buprenorphine, morphine, oxycodone, methadone, diamorphine

MECHANISM OF ACTION   Opioids act on opioid receptors (predominantly μ, but also ω and κ) in the CNS and peripheral nervous system, producing variable levels of agonism. These are G protein coupled receptors, which affect voltage–gated Ca^{2+} and K^+ channels, prolonging action potentials and thereby inhibiting neurotransmission in nociceptive pathways in the CNS. Tramadol acts on μ receptors but may also have noradrenergic and serotonergic effects.

INDICATIONS
- Moderate to severe pain
- Acute pulmonary oedema (diamorphine)

CAUTIONS AND CONTRA-INDICATIONS
- Acute respiratory depression
- Raised intracranial pressure
- Head injury
- Coma

SIDE-EFFECTS
- Nausea and vomiting
- Respiratory depression
- Hypotension
- Constipation
- Sedation and coma

METABOLISM AND HALF-LIFE   Opioids are metabolised by the liver. Codeine is a prodrug which is metabolised to morphine and other metabolites. About 8% of Caucasians lack CYP2D6 activity for codeine and, therefore, derive less analgesic benefit. $t_{1/2}$ varies: codeine 3–4 h; tramadol 6 h; fentanyl 7 h; morphine 2–3 h.

MONITORING   Monitor oxygen saturations and respiratory rate.

DRUG INTERACTIONS
- MAOIs may potentiate the action of morphine
- Use of CNS depressants (alcohol, sedatives, hypnotics, general anaesthetics) with opioids can increase the risk of side-effects, particularly respiratory depression

IMPORTANT POINTS
- Naloxone can be used to reverse the effects of opioids (coma, respiratory depression). It has a short duration of action and therefore repeated doses may be required
- Opioid analgesia can be combined with NSAIDs for effective analgesia – refer to the World Health Organization's Analgesic Ladder
- Opioids administered via epidurals or PCA devices can be used for the management of post-operative pain
- Repeated use of opioids may lead to dependence and tolerance
- When prescribing opioids also consider prescribing an anti-emetic and laxative
- Diamorphine has venodilatory effects, which reduce preload of the heart thereby reducing pulmonary oedema formation. It is also an anxiolytic
- Methadone is used during heroin withdrawal

Other antiepileptics

MECHANISM OF ACTION

Lamotrigine – stabilises inactive Na^+ channels thereby blocking repetitive firing of neurones and inhibiting the release of glutamate (which plays a key role in the generation of seizures).

Levetiracetam – exact mechanism is unclear. Effects may be mediated via blocking exocytosis of neurotransmitters and reduction of intraneuronal Ca^{2+} levels.

Topiramate – inhibits voltage-gated Na^+ channels and augments the activity of GABA at some subtypes of GABA receptors.

INDICATIONS
- Partial seizures with or without secondary generalisation (as monotherapy or adjunct)
- Generalised tonic–clonic seizures (as monotherapy or adjunct)
- Prophylaxis of migraine (topiramate)

CAUTIONS AND CONTRA-INDICATIONS
- Hypersensitivity
- Breastfeeding

SIDE-EFFECTS
- Hypersensitivity syndrome (most commonly with lamotrigine)
- GI disturbance
- Dizziness, ataxia, drowsiness and headaches
- Visual disturbance (acute myopia and choroidal effusions have been reported with topiramate)
- Confusion and rarely psychosis
- Rarely bone marrow failure

METABOLISM AND HALF-LIFE   Variable – e.g. lamotrigine ($t_{1/2}$ $\sim$33 h) is metabolised by the liver; levetiracetam ($t_{1/2}$ $\sim$7 h) is excreted largely unchanged in urine.

MONITORING   No specific drug monitoring required.

DRUG INTERACTIONS
- Reduced anticonvulsant effect with antidepressants
- Plasma concentrations may be affected by concomitant use of other antiepileptics
- Reduced contraceptive effect of OCP with topiramate

IMPORTANT POINTS
- Abrupt withdrawal can increase the risk of seizures
- Lamotrigine can cause Stevens–Johnson syndrome, particularly in children

Other antiparkinsonian drugs

MECHANISM OF ACTION

Dopamine D_2 receptor agonists (e.g. ergot-derived – bromocriptine, cabergoline; non-ergot-derived – ropinirole) – direct stimulation of dopamine receptors thereby countering the nigrostriatal dopamine deficiency in Parkinson's disease.

Catechol-O-methyltransferase (COMT) inhibitors (e.g. entacapone) – prevent the peripheral breakdown of L-dopa to methyldopa by COMT thereby increasing the amount of L-dopa available to the brain.

MAO-B inhibitors (e.g. selegiline) (see Monoamine oxidase inhibitors, p.54).

INDICATIONS
- Parkinson's disease
- Restless legs syndrome
- Hyperprolactinaemia (bromocriptine and cabergoline)

CAUTIONS AND CONTRA-INDICATIONS
- History of fibrotic disorders (dopamine receptor agonists)
- Phaeochromocytoma (COMT inhibitors)
- Caution in cardiac disease
- Caution in patients with a history of psychosis

SIDE-EFFECTS
- Nausea and vomiting
- Dopamine receptor agonists
  - Drowsiness and sudden onset of sleep
  - Dyskinesias
  - Hallucinations
  - Marked hypotension
- Fibrotic reactions (including pulmonary, retroperitoneal and pericardial fibrosis) (ergot-derived dopamine receptor agonists)
- Hepatic dysfunction (COMT inhibitors)
- Suppression of lactation (bromocriptine and cabergoline)

METABOLISM AND HALF-LIFE   Highly variable $t_{1/2}$; most are extensively metabolised.

MONITORING   Check chest x-ray, ESR, pulmonary function tests and serum creatinine prior to starting ergot-derived dopamine agonists; subsequently clinical monitoring for features of fibrosis is required. Monitor LFTs during treatment with COMT inhibitors.

DRUG INTERACTIONS
- Dopamine receptor agonists antagonised by antipsychotics and dopamine antagonist anti-emetics
- COMT inhibitors enhance anticoagulant effect of warfarin and enhance effects of sympathomimetics

IMPORTANT POINTS
- Dopamine receptor agonists may be used alone or as adjuncts to L-dopa. COMT inhibitors are used as adjuncts. Both groups may also be of benefit for patients experiencing severe 'end-of-dose' motor fluctuations
- Treatment should not be withdrawn abruptly

Paracetamol

MECHANISM OF ACTION   Weak anti-inflammatory activity through inhibition of COX enzymes and subsequent reduction in prostaglandin synthesis. Precise mechanism of antipyretic effect is poorly understood.

INDICATIONS
- Mild to moderate pain
- Pyrexia

CAUTIONS AND CONTRA-INDICATIONS
- Hypersensitivity
- Caution in hepatic impairment

SIDE-EFFECTS
- Rarely, rash or blood disorders

METABOLISM AND HALF-LIFE   Primarily metabolised in the liver by conjugation to glucuronide and sulphate. $t_{1/2}$ is ~2 h.

MONITORING   No specific drug monitoring required.

DRUG INTERACTIONS
- In overdose, increased risk of hepatotoxicity with hepatic enzyme inducers (e.g. chronic alcohol use, antiepileptics). Therefore a lower threshold for treatment with N-acetyl-cysteine should be used

IMPORTANT POINTS
- Paracetamol is the drug most commonly taken in overdose
- The amount of drug ingested should be calculated according to the patient's weight; doses of <150 mg/kg are unlikely to result in significant liver damage. Doses of >250 mg/kg carry a significant risk of hepatocellular toxicity and doses totalling >12 g are potentially fatal
- Paracetamol levels should be taken at least 4 h after ingestion
- Treatment with N-acetylcysteine should be commenced if levels exceed the treatment line on the paracetamol normogram
- For maximum protection N-acetylcysteine should be started within 8 h; if the overdose was taken more than 8 h previously or levels will not be available at 8 h after ingestion, treatment should commence immediately

Phenothiazine anti-emetics

EXAMPLES Prochlorperazine, chlorpromazine, promethazine

MECHANISM OF ACTION Mixed antagonists at muscarinic, histaminergic, dopaminergic, serotonergic and adrenergic receptors. Anti-emetic effect through inhibition of medullary CTZ. Also cause indirect reduction of stimuli to the brain stem reticular activating system, resulting in sedation hence use as typical antipsychotics.

INDICATIONS
- Severe nausea and vomiting
- Vertigo
- Labyrinthine disorders
- Psychotic disorders

CAUTIONS AND CONTRA-INDICATIONS
- CNS depression/coma
- Severe cardiovascular disease
- Caution in patients with hepatic impairment

SIDE-EFFECTS
- Sedation or agitation
- Extra-pyramidal symptoms (e.g. parkinsonian features, dystonia, akathisia, tardive dyskinesia)
- Postural hypotension
- Cardiac arrhythmias (prolongation of QT interval)
- Rarely transient jaundice

METABOLISM AND HALF-LIFE Metabolised in liver. $t_{1/2}$ highly variable – 8–35 h for chlorpromazine; 6–7 h for prochlorperazine.

MONITORING Monitor clinically for adverse effects.

DRUG INTERACTIONS
- Phenothiazines may enhance the CNS depressant effect of opioids, anxiolytics, sedatives, hypnotics and alcohol
- Antagonism of sympathomimetics, anticholinergics and antiepileptic drugs may occur (the latter may lower seizure threshold)
- Enhanced hypotensive effect with antihypertensive agents
- Increased risk of cardiac arrhythmias (including torsades de pointes) with other drugs that prolong the QT interval

IMPORTANT POINTS
- Phenothiazine anti-emetics are usually reserved for the treatment of nausea and vomiting that has not responded to pharmacotherapies targeting specific receptors, for example in PONV or in pregnancy

Phenytoin

MECHANISM OF ACTION Use-dependent blockade of voltage-dependent Na^+ channels responsible for the propagation of the action potential. They preferentially block the excitation of neurones that are repeatedly firing and therefore interrupt seizures.

INDICATIONS
- Epilepsy (not absence seizures)
- Trigeminal neuralgia
- Status epilepticus

CAUTIONS AND CONTRA-INDICATIONS
- Hypersensitivity
- Sinus bradycardia
- SA node block
- Second and third degree heart block
- Pregnancy

SIDE-EFFECTS
- GI disturbance
- Acne
- Insomnia
- Gingival hypertrophy
- Coarse facies
- Transient nervousness

METABOLISM AND HALF-LIFE Extensively metabolised by the liver. Exhibits zero-order kinetics.

MONITORING BP and cardiac monitoring is required when phenytoin is administered IV for status epilepticus. Plasma levels can be monitored when adjusting doses, to avoid toxicity.

DRUG INTERACTIONS
- Plasma levels are increased by macrolides, isoniazid, diltiazem and amiodarone
- Plasma levels are reduced by rifampicin and theophyllines
- Acute alcohol ingestion can increase phenytoin levels
- Chronic alcohol use can reduce phenytoin levels
- Warfarin levels can be affected by concomitant use of phenytoin
- Phenytoin reduces the effects of OCP and corticosteroids

IMPORTANT POINTS
- Risk of teratogenicity therefore avoid in pregnancy, as can predispose to neural tube defects and haemorrhagic disease of the newborn
- Narrow therapeutic index: careful monitoring with increasing doses
- Signs of toxicity include ataxia, slurred speech and nystagmus

Selective serotonin reuptake inhibitors (SSRIs)

EXAMPLES   Sertraline, paroxetine, fluoxetine

MECHANISM OF ACTION   The monoamine hypothesis postulates that impairment in central monoaminergic function with deficiencies in neurotransmitters (including 5-HT) are key to the aetiology of depression. SSRIs act to increase concentrations of 5-HT by preventing the reuptake of 5-HT back into the pre-synaptic terminal; they block specific 5-HT transporters thereby increasing 5-HT binding at the post-synaptic receptors.

INDICATIONS
- Depression
- Panic disorder
- Obsessive–compulsive disorder
- Generalised anxiety disorder

CAUTIONS AND CONTRA-INDICATIONS
- SSRIs should not be used in patients who suffer depression with active or recurrent episodes of mania

SIDE-EFFECTS
- GI disturbance
- Hypersensitivity reactions
- Anorexia and weight loss
- Dry mouth
- Headaches
- Sexual dysfunction

METABOLISM AND HALF-LIFE   Fluoxetine is primarily metabolised by the liver to the active metabolite norfluoxetine. Majority of SSRIs have a $t_{1/2}$ ranging from 15–24 h. Fluoxetine has a longer $t_{1/2}$.

MONITORING   No specific drug monitoring required.

DRUG INTERACTIONS
- SSRIs increase plasma concentrations of some TCAs
- Increased risk of convulsions when given with antiepileptics
- Risk of bleeding with aspirin, warfarin and NSAIDs
- Increased risk of serotonin syndrome with MAOIs

IMPORTANT POINTS
- It may take 2–4 weeks before patients notice a therapeutic benefit
- Due to irreversible MAO inhibition, SSRIs should not be started for at least 2 weeks after stopping MAOIs
- SSRIs should be withdrawn slowly due to the risk of rebound depression
- Use of SSRIs (e.g. paroxetine, sertraline) has been linked with suicidal ideation
- Patients should be reviewed every 1–2 weeks for at least 4 weeks until benefit is noticed. Treatment should continue for at least 6 months. Patients with recurrent depression should continue treatment for 2 years
- Serotonin syndrome may present with agitation, sweating, pyrexia, dilated pupils, tachycardia and high BP

Sodium valproate

MECHANISM OF ACTION Enhances the inhibitory effects of GABA within the brain, by inhibiting enzymes that inactivate GABA and block GABA reuptake into neurones. This leads to inhibition of action potential transmission both pre- and post-synaptically, thereby interrupting seizure activity.

INDICATIONS
- Epilepsy – all forms

CAUTIONS AND CONTRA-INDICATIONS
- Active liver disease
- Family history of severe liver disease
- Porphyria

SIDE-EFFECTS
- GI disturbance
- Weight gain
- Drowsiness
- Thrombocytopenia
- Rarely pancreatitis
- Hyperammonaemia
- Reduced bone mineral density
- Rarely liver dysfunction (including fatal hepatic failure)

METABOLISM AND HALF-LIFE Extensively metabolised by the liver; $t_{1/2}$ is 8–20 h.

MONITORING Monitor LFTs (6 monthly) and FBC (prior to commencing treatment and before surgical procedures).

DRUG INTERACTIONS
- Anticonvulsant effect reduced by antidepressants (SSRIs, TCAs), antimalarials (mefloquine, chloroquine) and MAOIs

IMPORTANT POINTS
- Risk of teratogenicity (including neural tube defects) if taken during pregnancy
- Serum valproate levels can be used to monitor compliance

Tricyclic antidepressants (TCAs)

EXAMPLES   Amitriptyline, lofepramine, imipramine, dosulepin

MECHANISM OF ACTION   Inhibit re-uptake of noradrenaline and serotonin into neurones, hence increasing synaptic availability of noradrenaline and serotonin. The increased extra-cellular concentration of neurotransmitters allows greater action potential transmission, leading to clinical improvement in symptoms.

INDICATIONS
- Depression
- Panic disorder
- Neuralgia
- Nocturnal enuresis in children

CAUTIONS AND CONTRA-INDICATIONS
- Immediately post-MI
- Cardiac arrhythmias
- In manic phase of bipolar disorder
- Severe liver disease

SIDE-EFFECTS
- Arrhythmias
- Anxiety
- Dizziness
- Drowsiness
- Antimuscarinic effects (e.g. dry mouth, blurred vision, constipation, urinary retention)

METABOLISM AND HALF-LIFE   Metabolised in the liver; $t_{1/2}$ is 9–25 h.

MONITORING   No specific drug monitoring required.

DRUG INTERACTIONS
- Should not be given with MAOIs due to risk of hypertensive crisis and hyperpyrexia
- Other antidepressants should be prescribed with consideration of the mechanism and effects of co-administration
- Increased sedative effect when taken with alcohol and antihistamines
- Increased antimuscarinic side-effects when taken with antihistamines and anticholinergics
- TCAs reduce seizure threshold and antagonise the effects of antiepileptic medication

IMPORTANT POINTS
- When taken in overdose can be fatal due to cardiac arrhythmias (ECG changes include sinus tachycardia, prolonged PR interval, prolonged QRS duration, prolonged QT interval and non-specific ST- and T-wave changes)
- TCAs have varying sedative properties (sedating – amitriptyline, dosulepin; non-sedating – lofepramine, imipramine), which may affect ability to drive
- There may be a delay of up to 2 weeks after starting treatment with TCAs before symptomatic improvement is seen

Aciclovir

MECHANISM OF ACTION   Synthetic analogue of guanosine, which is phosphorylated to become an active compound, aciclovir triphosphate. Aciclovir triphosphate competes with the natural nucleotide as a substrate to viral DNA polymerase and thus inhibits viral DNA replication.

INDICATIONS
- Treatment and prophylaxis of herpes simplex infections
- Treatment of herpes zoster and varicella infections

CAUTIONS AND CONTRA-INDICATIONS
- Hypersensitivity to aciclovir
- Caution in renal impairment (dose adjustment may be required)

SIDE-EFFECTS
- GI disturbance
- Headache and dizziness
- Rash
- Fatigue
- Fever
- Renal failure

METABOLISM AND HALF-LIFE $t_{1/2}$ is between 2.5–3 h. Most of the drug is excreted unchanged in urine.

MONITORING   Regular monitoring of renal function is required in elderly patients on long-term or IV therapy.

DRUG INTERACTIONS
- Increased risk of nephrotoxicity with concomitant use of ciclosporin or tacrolimus

IMPORTANT POINTS
- Maintain adequate hydration in patients on high doses or with renal failure (to reduce the risk of nephrotoxicity)
- Elderly patients are at risk of neurological reactions due to reduced renal function and hence clearance. Examples of neurological symptoms include agitation, confusion, tremor, ataxia, convulsions and encephalopathy
- IV treatment for 10 days is usually required for encephalitis
- Can be given topically for skin and eye disease

Aminoglycosides

EXAMPLES   Gentamicin, tobramycin, amikacin, neomycin, streptomycin

MECHANISM OF ACTION   Bacteriocidal antibiotic that blocks protein synthesis by binding to the bacterial 30S ribosomal subunit. This prevents the process of tRNA attachment and mRNA translation is disrupted.

INDICATIONS
- Septicaemia
- Biliary tract infection
- Acute pyelonephritis and prostatitis
- Endocarditis
- Adjunct in *Listeria* meningitis

CAUTIONS AND CONTRA-INDICATIONS
- Myasthenia gravis (aminoglycosides can impair neurotransmission within muscles)
- Caution in renal failure (doses should be reduced)

SIDE-EFFECTS
- GI disturbance
- Nephrotoxicity
- Rash
- Vestibular and auditory damage (ototoxicity)
- Blood dyscrasias

METABOLISM AND HALF-LIFE   Aminoglycosides are excreted unchanged in the urine. $t_{1/2}$ for gentamicin is 2–3 h.

MONITORING   Regular monitoring of U&Es. For single daily dosing, gentamicin level must be taken 6–12 h after the first dose. Levels should be interpreted using the Hartford Nomogram, which will determine dosing frequency.

DRUG INTERACTIONS
- Increased risk of ototoxicity with loop diuretics
- Aminoglycosides can enhance the effects of non-depolarising muscle relaxants
- Increased risk of nephrotoxicity with ciclosporin

IMPORTANT POINTS
- Predominantly Gram-negative *Enterobacteria* spp. cover (e.g. UTI, abdominal sepsis) and *Pseudomonas* spp.
- Poor oral absorption hence given parenterally (except neomycin)
- Once daily aminoglycoside dosing is preferable and provides adequate serum concentrations. Exceptions include the treatment of bacterial endocarditis
- Continuation of gentamicin therapy for more than 7 days carries an increased risk of nephrotoxicity and ototoxicity

Antifungals

MECHANISM OF ACTION

Polyene antifungals (e.g. nystatin, amphotericin) – bind to the cell membrane and interfere with ionic permeability and transport.

Azole antifungals (ketoconazole, itraconazole, fluconazole) – inhibit fungal cell wall ergosterol synthesis, which affects membrane enzymes and cell replication.

Griseofulvin – fungistatic agent that binds to tubulin and interferes with microtubule formation, thereby preventing mitosis; also interferes with hyphal cell wall synthesis.

Terbinafine – allylamine which interferes with fungal sterol biosynthesis by inhibiting squalene epoxidase, ultimately leading to fungal cell death.

INDICATIONS
- Oral, skin and vaginal candidiasis (polyenes, azoles)
- Dermatophyte infections (terbinafine, griseofulvin)
- Histoplasmosis (azoles, polyenes)
- Aspergillosis infections (polyenes, azoles)
- Cryptococcal meningitis (polyenes, azoles)

CAUTIONS AND CONTRA-INDICATIONS
- Hypersensitivity
- Caution in renal and hepatic impairment (may require dose adjustment)
- Pregnancy and breastfeeding (griseofulvin, ketoconazole)
- SLE (griseofulvin may exacerbate symptoms)

SIDE-EFFECTS
- Anorexia and GI disturbance
- Muscle and joint pain
- Rash and pruritus
- Headache
- Hepatotoxicity (azole antifungals)

METABOLISM AND HALF-LIFE $t_{1/2}$ for amphotericin is $\sim$170 h; $t_{1/2}$ for ketoconazole is $\sim$8 h; $t_{1/2}$ for fluconazole is $\sim$25 h; itraconazole is extensively metabolised in the liver and $t_{1/2}$ is $\sim$36 h.

MONITORING   Monitor LFTs with itraconazole and ketoconazole.

DRUG INTERACTIONS
- Itraconazole can precipitate heart failure if given in high doses and for long periods to elderly patients or individuals with IHD/prescribed negative inotropes (e.g. CCBs)
- Amphotericin can result in renal impairment when administered with other nephrotoxic drugs
- The dose of terbinafine may need to be adjusted with co-administration of drugs that are metabolised via Cytochrome P450

IMPORTANT POINTS
- Amphotericin is administered IV to treat systemic fungal infections
- Nystatin is available in topical and oral preparations to treat candidiasis
- Terbinafine is commonly used to treat fungal nail infections

Antiretroviral agents

MECHANISM OF ACTION

NRTIs (e.g. zidovudine, lamivudine) – nucleoside analogues which terminate elongation of DNA chains, thereby inhibiting synthesis of viral DNA from the RNA genome.

NNRTIs (e.g. nevirapine) – allosteric inhibition of reverse transcriptase, causing a conformational change and subsequent inactivation.

Protease inhibitors (e.g. saquinavir) – inhibit post-translational modification of viral polypeptides, thereby preventing assembly of viral components.

INDICATIONS

- HIV infection
- Prevention of mother to child transmission (zidovudine)
- Post-HIV exposure prophylaxis
- Chronic hepatitis B infection (lamivudine)

CAUTIONS AND CONTRA-INDICATIONS

- Caution in hepatic impairment (NRTIs may cause potentially life-threatening lactic acidosis in patients with liver disease)
- Caution in renal impairment or pre-existing haematological conditions

SIDE-EFFECTS

- GI disturbance
- Hepatotoxicity
- Blood disorders (including anaemia, neutropenia and thrombocytopenia)
- Pancreatitis
- Peripheral neuropathy (NRTIs)
- Hypersensitivity reactions
- Osteonecrosis
- Lipodystrophy syndrome (insulin resistance, fat redistribution and dyslipidaemia)

METABOLISM AND HALF-LIFE   Metabolism, elimination and $t_{1/2}$ vary within and between classes.

MONITORING   Check CD4$^+$ cell count, viral load, LFTs and for adverse clinical features.

DRUG INTERACTIONS

- Concomitant treatment with potentially nephrotoxic or myelosuppressive drugs may increase the risk of adverse effects

IMPORTANT POINTS

- The aim of treatment is to reduce viral load as much as possible, for as long as possible; it should be initiated and supervised by a specialist mindful of the potential adverse drug reactions
- Development of drug resistance is a common problem but is reduced by using a combination of drugs with synergistic or additive effects
- Post-exposure prophylaxis may be appropriate; in the event of exposure to HIV-contaminated materials local and national guidelines should be followed
- Use of antiretrovirals during pregnancy and labour can significantly reduce mother to child transmission of HIV

Antituberculosis drugs

MECHANISM OF ACTION

Ethambutol – precise mechanism of action is unclear; may disrupt cell wall formation by preventing incorporation of mycolic acids.

Isoniazid – inhibits synthesis of lipid constituents of the bacterial cell wall.

Pyrazinamide – prodrug converted to pyrazinoic acid at low pH, however, the precise mechanism of action is unclear.

Rifampicin – inhibits synthesis of bacterial RNA via inhibition of DNA-dependent RNA polymerase.

Streptomycin – binds to bacterial 30S ribosomal subunit to inhibit protein synthesis.

INDICATIONS
- Tuberculosis
- Non-tuberculous mycobacterium infections

CAUTIONS AND CONTRA-INDICATIONS
- Caution in renal and hepatic impairment
- Caution in elderly and in hearing impairment (streptomycin)
- Pregnancy (streptomycin should not be used; caution with rifampicin and isoniazid)

SIDE-EFFECTS
- Hypersensitivity reactions
- Hepatotoxicity (isoniazid, rifampicin, pyrazinamide)
- Retrobulbar neuritis (ethambutol)
- Peripheral neuropathy (isoniazid)
- Hyperuricaemia and gout (pyrazinamide)
- Orange-red discolouration of urine and tears (rifampicin)
- 'Flu-like' symptoms and fever (rifampicin)
- Ototoxicity and nephrotoxicity (streptomycin)

METABOLISM AND HALF-LIFE $t_{1/2}$ variable. Ethambutol, isoniazid and streptomycin are excreted largely unchanged in urine. Rifampicin is mainly excreted via bile. Pyrazinamide is metabolised by the liver.

MONITORING   Check LFTs and U&Es prior to and during treatment. Visual acuity should be tested before and during treatment with ethambutol. Patients should be warned of possible side-effects and advised to seek immediate medical attention if signs of liver dysfunction occur.

DRUG INTERACTIONS
- Isoniazid increases plasma concentration of antiepileptics
- Rifampicin is a hepatic enzyme inducer (Cytochrome P450) that accelerates the metabolism of several drugs including oestrogens, corticosteroids, phenytoin and anticoagulants
- For interactions of streptomycin (see Aminoglycosides, p.66)

IMPORTANT POINTS
- Treatment should be initiated and managed by a specialist physician
- Pulmonary tuberculosis is usually treated in 2 phases (i.e. 2 months with 4 drugs and 4 further months with 2 drugs, usually rifampicin and isoniazid); regimens for extrapulmonary tuberculosis differ
- Compliance is frequently a problem; direct observed therapy may be considered

Cephalosporins and other β lactams

EXAMPLES First-generation cephalosporins – cefalexin, cefradine; second-generation cephalosporins – cefuroxime; third-generation cephalosporins – cefotaxime, ceftriaxone, ceftazidime; carbapenems – imipenem, ertapenem; piperacillin

MECHANISM OF ACTION Mechanism is similar to penicillins except that cephalosporins are relatively resistant to staphylococcal β lactamases. They penetrate the CSF poorly unless meningeal inflammation is present. Piperacillin when combined with tazobactam (a β lactamase inhibitor) has good activity against *Pseudomonas* spp.

INDICATIONS
- Pneumonia
- Sepsis
- Biliary tract infection
- UTI
- Peritonitis
- Meningitis

CAUTIONS AND CONTRA-INDICATIONS
- Hypersensitivity
- Caution in renal impairment (dose adjustment required)

SIDE-EFFECTS
- Urticarial rash
- Anaphylaxis
- GI disturbance
- Stevens–Johnson syndrome
- Cholestatic jaundice (ceftriaxone)
- Antibiotic-associated colitis

METABOLISM AND HALF-LIFE Excreted via the kidneys. $t_{1/2}$ for cefotaxime is $\sim$1 h; $t_{1/2}$ for ceftriaxone is 6–9 h. $t_{1/2}$ for imipenem is $\sim$1 h. $t_{1/2}$ for piperacillin–tazobactam is 36–72 min.

MONITORING No specific drug monitoring required.

DRUG INTERACTIONS
- Reduced efficacy of the OCP when taking cephalosporins. Women should be warned of this and advised to use alternative contraceptive methods

IMPORTANT POINTS
- Piperacillin combined with tazobactam (Tazocin®) may be used in the treatment of neutropenic sepsis. It is being increasingly used in immunocompetent hosts for resistant infections and for pseudomonal infection
- 10% of patients who are hypersensitive to penicillins may have a similar reaction to cephalosporins and other β lactams

Penicillins

EXAMPLES (in order of narrowest to broadest spectrum) Standard penicillins – benzyl-penicillin, phenoxymethylpenicillin; antistaphylococcal penicillins – flucloxacillin; amino-penicillins – ampicillin, amoxicillin

MECHANISM OF ACTION   β lactam moiety binds to and inhibits the transpeptidase required for the formation of peptidoglycan cross-links within the bacterial cell wall. This results in defective bacterial cell wall synthesis and subsequent cytolysis. Flucloxacillin is relatively resistant to staphylococcal β lactamases. Aminopenicillins have enhanced activity against aerobic Gram-negative bacilli. Co-amoxiclav is a combination of amoxicillin and clavulanic acid (a β lactamase inhibitor).

INDICATIONS
- Pharyngitis/tonsillitis
- Pneumonia
- Otitis media
- Cellulitis
- Meningitis
- Endocarditis
- Rheumatic fever
- Osteomyelitis
- UTI

CAUTIONS AND CONTRA-INDICATIONS
- Hypersensitivity

SIDE-EFFECTS
- Urticarial rash
- Anaphylaxis
- GI disturbance
- Antibiotic-associated colitis
- Stevens–Johnson syndrome
- Fever
- Joint pains
- Rarely cholestatic jaundice with flucloxacillin or co-amoxiclav

METABOLISM AND HALF-LIFE   Elimination is via the kidneys and biliary tract. $t_{1/2}$ for benzylpenicillin is ~30 min; $t_{1/2}$ for flucloxacillin is ~50 min; $t_{1/2}$ for amoxicillin is ~1 h.

MONITORING   No specific drug monitoring required.

DRUG INTERACTIONS
- Reduced efficacy of the OCP when taking penicillins. Women should be warned of this and advised to use alternative contraceptive methods

IMPORTANT POINTS
- Benzylpenicillin (penicillin G) must be administered parenterally because it is inactivated by gastric acid secretions; phenoxymethylpenicillin (penicillin V) has a similar spectrum of activity to benzylpenicillin but can be administered orally
- Patients with infectious mononucleosis may get a diffuse, erythematous, maculopapular rash when treated with ampicillin or amoxicillin

Glycopeptide antibiotics

EXAMPLES Vancomycin, teicoplanin

MECHANISM OF ACTION Inhibit bacterial cell wall synthesis by sterically and irreversibly blocking the elongation of peptidoglycan chains. The activity of glycopeptides is bactericidal.

INDICATIONS
- Gram-positive infections (including methicillin-resistant staphylococci and penicillin-resistant pneumococci)
- Prophylaxis and treatment of endocarditis
- Antibiotic-associated colitis due to *Clostridium difficile*

CAUTIONS AND CONTRA-INDICATIONS
- Hypersensitivity
- Caution in renal impairment (may require dose reduction)
- Caution in inflammatory disorders of the intestinal mucosa due to increased systemic absorption with oral dosing and thus increased risk of adverse effects
- Hearing loss or susceptibility to auditory damage

SIDE-EFFECTS
- Nephrotoxicity
- Ototoxicity (including hearing loss and tinnitus)
- Fevers and chills
- Hypersensitivity reactions
- Neutropenia
- Thrombophlebitis at infusion site if administered IV

METABOLISM AND HALF-LIFE Excreted unchanged by kidney; $t_{1/2}$ is 3–6 h.

MONITORING Pre-dose (trough) plasma levels should be checked prior to third or fourth dose of vancomycin after initiation or change in dose. Monitor FBC and U&Es. Also consider monitoring auditory function in children, elderly or in renal impairment. Teicoplanin levels are not routinely monitored.

DRUG INTERACTIONS
- Caution with other ototoxic or nephrotoxic agents

IMPORTANT POINTS
- Glycopeptides are unable to penetrate the cell membrane of Gram-negative bacteria due to their high molecular weight. Therefore, their spectrum of activity comprises aerobic and anaerobic Gram-positive organisms (including *Staphylococcus* spp., *Streptococcus* spp. and *Enterococcus* spp.)
- Systemic absorption of oral glycopeptides is poor, however, the enteral route is used for the treatment of *C. difficile* colitis
- Glycopeptides are very irritant. Parenteral vancomycin must be administered IV due to injection site necrosis with IM route; this is less problematic with teicoplanin, which can be administered IM. Additionally, IV infusion sites should be rotated to minimise local irritation
- Vancomycin may cause release of histamine when infused rapidly, resulting in a diffuse erythematous rash ('red man syndrome')

Macrolides

EXAMPLES   Erythromycin, azithromycin, clarithromycin

MECHANISM OF ACTION   Inhibition of bacterial RNA-dependent protein synthesis by reversibly binding to the 50S subunit of ribosomes within the organism. This affects bacterial growth and may be either bacteriostatic or bacteriocidal.

INDICATIONS
- Respiratory tract infections
- Campylobacter enteritis
- Urethritis (non-gonococcal)
- Pertussis infection
- Skin and soft tissue infections
- Otitis media
- *Helicobacter pylori* eradication

CAUTIONS AND CONTRA-INDICATIONS
- Liver disease
- Hypersensitivity

SIDE-EFFECTS
- Nausea and vomiting
- Diarrhoea
- Hepatitis
- Anorexia
- Pancreatitis
- Headaches

METABOLISM AND HALF-LIFE   Metabolised in the liver and excreted via the biliary route. $t_{1/2}$ is variable – $t_{1/2}$ for erythromycin is 1–1.5 h; $t_{1/2}$ for azithromycin is 2–4 days; $t_{1/2}$ for clarithromycin is 3–7 h.

MONITORING   No specific drug monitoring required.

DRUG INTERACTIONS
- Enhanced anticoagulant effect of warfarin
- Macrolides inhibit the metabolism of theophylline, thereby increasing plasma levels
- Increased plasma levels of carbamazepine with concomitant use of macrolides
- Increased risk of cardiac arrhythmias with amiodarone due to QT prolongation

IMPORTANT POINTS
- Erythromycin has similar bacterial sensitivity to penicillins and therefore can be used as an alternative in penicillin allergic patients
- *Helicobacter pylori* eradication therapy consists of 2 antibiotics and a PPI. Current guidance suggest 1 week of either amoxicillin or metronidazole and clarithromycin and a PPI
- Macrolides are effective against community-acquired pneumonia caused by atypical organisms (*Mycoplasma* spp., *Chlamydia* spp., *Legionella* spp.)

Metronidazole

MECHANISM OF ACTION   Precise mechanism of action is unclear, however, metronidazole possesses a nitro-group that becomes charged and trapped within the intracellular compartment of anaerobes. This leads to bacterial DNA damage and ultimately strand breakage and subsequent cell death.

INDICATIONS
- Surgical prophylaxis
- Anaerobic infections (including dental and abdominal sepsis)
- Aspiration pneumonia
- Protozoal infections
- Pelvic inflammatory disease

CAUTIONS AND CONTRA-INDICATIONS
- Known hypersensitivity to metronidazole

SIDE-EFFECTS
- GI disturbance
- Metallic taste in mouth
- Anorexia
- Rarely hepatitis
- Pancreatitis
- Peripheral neuropathy (with prolonged therapy)

METABOLISM AND HALF-LIFE $t_{1/2}$ is ~8.5 h. Metabolised to active compounds by the liver with 75% excreted in urine.

MONITORING   No specific drug monitoring required.

DRUG INTERACTIONS
- Alcohol should be avoided while taking metronidazole (see below)
- Concomitant use of ciclosporin can lead to elevated ciclosporin serum levels
- Possible potentiation of anticoagulant therapy has been reported when metronidazole is used with warfarin

IMPORTANT POINTS
- Metronidazole is a potent inhibitor of obligate anaerobes and protozoa such as *Trichomonas* spp. and *Entamoeba* spp.
- Patients should be advised to completely avoid alcohol during and for 48 h after a course of metronidazole due to the risk of a severe disulfiram-like reaction (flushing and hypotension)
- Metronidazole can be used in chronic renal failure; however, it is rapidly removed from plasma by dialysis

Nitrofurantoin

MECHANISM OF ACTION The precise mechanism of action is poorly understood; reactive nitrofurantoin metabolites damage a number of macromolecules within bacterial cells including ribosomal proteins and DNA. Nitrofurantoin is bactericidal and is active against most urinary pathogens, including *Escherichia coli*, *Enterococcus faecalis*, *Klebsiella* spp., and *Staphylococcus* spp. (including *S. aureus*, *S. saprophyticus* and *S. epidermidis*).

INDICATIONS
- Uncomplicated UTI

CAUTIONS AND CONTRA-INDICATIONS
- Renal impairment
- Pregnant patients at term and infants under 3 months (due to the risk of haemolytic anaemia in the neonate)
- Caution in conditions associated with peripheral neuropathy (due to potentially severe and irreversible neuronal adverse affects)

SIDE-EFFECTS
- GI disturbance
- Peripheral neuropathy
- Hypersensitivity reactions
- Pulmonary fibrosis (if prolonged use)
- Haemolytic anaemia
- Hepatic dysfunction

METABOLISM AND HALF-LIFE $t_{1/2}$ is ~30 min. Approximately 40% is excreted unchanged in the urine and the remainder is rapidly metabolised by tissues.

MONITORING No specific drug monitoring required.

DRUG INTERACTIONS
- Absorption of nitrofurantoin may be reduced by magnesium-containing antacids
- Antibacterial effects of nitrofurantoin antagonised by quinolones

IMPORTANT POINTS
- In uncomplicated UTI in females a 3-day course is usually adequate
- Nitrofurantoin should not be used if there is a possibility of bacteraemia because plasma concentrations of the drug are low
- Nitrofurantoin is ineffective against *Proteus* spp. because its activity is reduced in alkaline pH (as created by the ammonium-producing urease enzyme of *Proteus* bacteria); also ineffective against *Pseudomonas* spp.

Quinolones

EXAMPLES Ciprofloxacin, levofloxacin, ofloxacin

MECHANISM OF ACTION The bactericidal action of ciprofloxacin results from the inhibition of both type II (DNA gyrase) and type IV topoisomerases, required for bacterial DNA replication, transcription, repair and recombination.

INDICATIONS
- UTI
- Infections of the GI system
- Bronchopulmonary infections
- Typhoid fever
- Gonorrhoea and non-gonococcal urethritis and cervicitis
- Anthrax

CAUTIONS AND CONTRA-INDICATIONS
- Patients with a history of tendon disorders related to quinolones
- Pregnancy, children and growing adolescents (due to the risk of joint arthropathy)
- Avoid in patients with CNS disorders (e.g. epilepsy – can reduce seizure threshold)

SIDE-EFFECTS
- GI disturbance
- Headaches
- Dizziness
- Rashes (including Stevens–Johnson syndrome)
- Tendon inflammation and damage
- Confusion, anxiety and depression
- Phototoxicity with excessive sunlight
- Seizures

METABOLISM AND HALF-LIFE $t_{1/2}$ for ciprofloxacin is 3-6 h. Ciprofloxacin is excreted predominately unchanged in urine.

MONITORING No specific drug monitoring required.

DRUG INTERACTIONS
- Increased risk of nephrotoxicity when quinolones given with ciclosporin
- Possible increased risk of convulsions when quinolones given with NSAIDs or theophylline (also increases theophylline levels)
- Ciprofloxacin enhances anticoagulant effect of warfarin
- Increased risk of torsades de pointes with other drugs that also prolong the QT interval
- Reduced efficacy when given with aluminium- or magnesium-containing antacids or iron preparations

IMPORTANT POINTS
- Quinolones may impair performance of skilled tasks (e.g. driving); this effect is enhanced by alcohol
- Discontinue if psychiatric, neurological or hypersensitivity reactions (including severe rash) occur
- Ciprofloxacin is active against Gram-negative bacteria such as *Salmonella* spp., *Shigella* spp., *Campylobacter* spp., *Neisseria* spp. and *Pseudomonas* spp.

Tetracyclines

EXAMPLES   Doxycycline, tetracycline, oxytetracycline

MECHANISM OF ACTION   Active uptake into a susceptible organism results in inhibition of protein synthesis. Their bacteriostatic effect is achieved by binding to the prokaryotic 30S ribosomal subunit and inhibiting aminoacyl tRNA and mRNA ribosomal complex formation. Additionally, topical tetracyclines are used in the treatment of acne. This effect is mediated through inhibition of neutrophil activity and pro-inflammatory reactions, including those associated with phospholipase A_2, endogenous nitric oxide and interleukin-6.

INDICATIONS
- Urogenital tract infections (e.g. salpingitis, urethritis caused by *Chlamydia* spp.)
- LRTI (particularly *Haemophilus influenzae* infections in COPD patients)
- Acne vulgaris and rosacea

CAUTIONS AND CONTRA-INDICATIONS
- Hypersensitivity to tetracyclines
- Children under 12 (deposition in bone and teeth – risk of staining)
- Pregnancy and breastfeeding
- Acute porphyria
- Chronic kidney disease

SIDE-EFFECTS
- GI disturbance
- Dysphagia and oesophageal irritation
- Blood disorders
- Hypersensitivity reactions (including Stevens–Johnson syndrome)
- Photosensitivity

METABOLISM AND HALF-LIFE $t_{1/2}$ is variable depending on drug. Tetracyclines are concentrated by the liver in bile and excreted in urine and faeces at high concentrations in a biologically active form.

MONITORING   No specific monitoring required.

DRUG INTERACTIONS
- Tetracyclines can enhance the effects of warfarin (due to enzymatic inhibition)
- Risk of idiopathic intracranial hypertension when tetracyclines used with retinoids
- Doxycycline can increase plasma concentrations of ciclosporin

IMPORTANT POINTS
- Patients are advised to use high-factor sun protection and avoid direct sun exposure when on doxycycline (due to photosensitivity)
- Tetracyclines should be avoided in anyone taking potentially hepatotoxic drugs

Trimethoprim

MECHANISM OF ACTION   Binds to bacterial dihydrofolate reductase and irreversibly inhibits the production of tetrahydrofolate, which is a precursor for the synthesis of thymidine. This results in inhibition of bacterial DNA synthesis.

INDICATIONS
- UTI

CAUTIONS AND CONTRA-INDICATIONS
- Blood dyscrasias
- Caution in patients with renal impairment

SIDE-EFFECTS
- GI disturbance
- Pruritis
- Rashes
- Hyperkalaemia

METABOLISM AND HALF-LIFE   Approximately 50% is bound to plasma protein. $t_{1/2}$ ranges from 8.6–17 h. Elimination is via the kidneys.

MONITORING   No specific drug monitoring required.

DRUG INTERACTIONS
- Increased risk of ventricular arrhythmias with amiodarone
- Increased risk of nephrotoxicity when given with ciclosporin
- Increased risk of haematological toxicity when given with azathioprine and methotrexate

IMPORTANT POINTS
- Commonly sensitive organisms include Gram-positive aerobes (*Staphylococcus* spp.) and Gram-negative aerobes (*Enterobacter* spp., *Haemophilus* spp., *Klebsiella* spp.)
- Local policies should be consulted prior to prescribing antibiotics due to emerging resistance of organisms
- Co-trimoxazole is a combination of trimethoprim and sulfamethoxazole, which inhibits an earlier stage of tetrahydrofolate synthesis. It is the drug of choice in the treatment of *Pneumocystis jiroveci* pneumonia

5α-reductase inhibitors

EXAMPLES   Dutasteride, finasteride

MECHANISM OF ACTION   Competitively inhibit the metabolism of testosterone to dihydrotestosterone (a more potent androgen) in peripheral tissues. Reduced circulating dihydrotestosterone leads to reduced prostatic volume and thereby relief of voiding symptoms.

INDICATIONS
• Benign prostatic hyperplasia

CAUTIONS AND CONTRA-INDICATIONS
• Should not be given in women, children or adolescents
• Severe liver disease

SIDE-EFFECTS
• Impotence
• Decreased libido
• Ejaculation disorders
• Breast tenderness/enlargement

METABOLISM AND HALF-LIFE   Metabolised in the liver with the majority excreted via the GI tract. $t_{1/2}$ for dutasteride is 3–5 weeks (at therapeutic concentrations); $t_{1/2}$ for finasteride is 5–6 h (longer in patients >70 years).

MONITORING   No specific drug monitoring required.

DRUG INTERACTIONS
• Plasma levels of dutasteride may be increased if long-term administration with protease inhibitors (ritonavir, indinavir) or antifungals (ketoconazole, itraconazole)

IMPORTANT POINTS
• Finasteride can be used in combination with doxazosin (α blocker) to treat benign prostatic hyperplasia
• These drugs cause a reduction in serum PSA levels of ~50%. Therefore, interpretation of PSA levels should take this into account
• Women of childbearing potential should avoid handling broken tablets/capsules
• Patients may require several months treatment before a benefit is observed

Antidiuretic hormone (ADH) analogues

EXAMPLES   Vasopressin, terlipressin, desmopressin

MECHANISM OF ACTION   Effect on the kidney is mediated through stimulation of vasopressin (V_2) receptors, increasing water reabsorption in the collecting duct. Vasopressin (V_1) receptor binding, at higher concentrations, promotes vasoconstriction of vascular smooth muscle in the GI system (intestine, gallbladder) and urinary bladder. The action of ADH analogues on V_1 receptors also promotes factor VIII release from endothelial cells.

INDICATIONS
- Pituitary diabetes insipidus (vasopressin and desmopressin)
- Bleeding oesophageal varices (vasopressin and terlipressin)
- Haemophilia and von Willebrand disease (desmopressin)
- Primary nocturnal enuresis (desmopressin)

CAUTIONS AND CONTRA-INDICATIONS
- Coronary artery disease
- Chronic nephritis

SIDE-EFFECTS
- Fluid retention
- Pallor
- Tremor
- Vertigo
- Headaches
- Peripheral ischaemia
- GI disturbance (e.g. cramps)
- Hypersensitivity reactions (including anaphylaxis)
- Constriction of coronary arteries precipitating ischaemia

METABOLISM AND HALF-LIFE   Variable – e.g. vasopressin has a plasma $t_{1/2}$ of 10 min and its metabolism is via the liver and kidney; $t_{1/2}$ for desmopressin is dependent on route of administration (IN ~3.5 h, IV ~3 h, PO 2–3 h)

MONITORING   Intravenous use requires close monitoring of vital signs (i.e. BP, pulse). Serum U&Es should be monitored.

IMPORTANT POINTS
- Desmopressin has a longer duration of action and lacks vasoconstrictor properties hence is preferable to other ADH analogues
- Desmopressin is used in the water deprivation test to help distinguish between cranial and nephrogenic diabetes insipidus

Biguanides

EXAMPLES Metformin

MECHANISM OF ACTION Oral hypoglycaemic agent that increases glucose uptake and utilisation in skeletal muscle, hence reducing insulin resistance. Metformin also inhibits hepatic gluconeogenesis and glycogenolysis. It increases the transport capacity of all types of membrane GLUT and is only functional when endogenous insulin is present.

INDICATIONS
- Type 2 diabetes mellitus
- Polycystic ovarian syndrome (unlicensed)

CAUTIONS AND CONTRA-INDICATIONS
- Caution in renal impairment (avoid if eGFR <30 ml/min)
- Use of iodine-containing x-ray contrast media
- Ketoacidosis

SIDE-EFFECTS
- GI disturbance
- Taste disturbance (metallic taste)
- Lactic acidosis
- Erythema, pruritus and urticaria

METABOLISM AND HALF-LIFE $t_{1/2}$ for metformin is ~3 h and it is excreted unchanged in urine.

MONITORING Monitor renal function regularly (at least annually).

DRUG INTERACTIONS
- Increased risk of lactic acidosis with heavy alcohol intake
- Hypoglycaemic effects enhanced by ACEIs and MAOIs
- Hypoglycaemic effects antagonised by thiazide diuretics

IMPORTANT POINTS
- Metformin is used as a first-line agent in obese patients (due to appetite suppressant effect); it does not stimulate insulin release, hence poses no risk of inducing hypoglycaemia
- Metformin can be combined with other oral hypoglycaemic drugs and insulin if required
- Metformin can induce lactic acidosis in renal impairment
- Patients requiring contrast for radiological investigations should be advised not to restart metformin until renal function returns to normal
- Metformin should be withdrawn in patients susceptible to hypoxia or deteriorating renal function

Bisphosphonates

EXAMPLES   Alendronate, etidronate, pamidronate, risedronate

MECHANISM OF ACTION   Bisphosphonates are adsorbed onto bone surfaces, inhibiting bone resorption by osteoclasts and promoting apoptosis of osteoclasts in favour of osteoblast action and calcium uptake. This serves to prevent further reduction in bone mass.

INDICATIONS
- Prophylaxis and treatment of osteoporosis
- Paget's disease
- Hypercalaemia
- Bony metastases

CAUTIONS AND CONTRA-INDICATIONS
- Oesophageal abnormalities (e.g. strictures and motility disorders)
- Pregnancy

SIDE-EFFECTS
- Oesophageal irritation
- GI disturbance
- Melaena
- Flu-like symptoms
- Musculoskeletal pain
- Headache
- Hypocalcaemia

METABOLISM AND HALF-LIFE $t_{1/2}$ is ~1 h for pamidronate; other bisphosphonates have significantly longer half-lives due to high uptake into bone tissue.

MONITORING   Usually no specific drug monitoring is required but, if given for hypercalcaemia, serum calcium levels and clinical symptoms (tetany, paraesthesia) should be monitored.

DRUG INTERACTIONS
- Reduced absorption of bisphosphonates with antacids, calcium salts and iron supplements

IMPORTANT POINTS
- Frequency of administration is dependent on indication and drug
- For the treatment of osteoporosis, co-prescription of calcium and vitamin D is advised
- NICE guidance (October 2008) recommends alendronate as a treatment option for the secondary prevention of fragility fractures in post-menopausal women with confirmed osteoporosis
- Patients should be advised to take bisphosphonates on an empty stomach, 30 min before eating with plenty of water. They should remain sitting or standing upright for 30 min after taking the tablets (to avoid oesophageal irritation)
- Pamidronate can be administered IV in the treatment of acute hypercalcaemia
- The use of bisphosphonates (particularly administered IV and high potency) can result in osteonecrosis of the jaw. Oncology patients should have a dental assessment prior to receiving bisphosphonate therapy

Carbimazole

MECHANISM OF ACTION   A prodrug that undergoes metabolism to the active metabolite, thiamazole. The latter inhibits the iodination of tyrosyl residues in thyroglobulin. This is mediated through the enzyme thyroid peroxidase and it also inhibits the coupling of iodotyrosines. Both actions inhibit thyroid hormone production.

INDICATIONS
- Hyperthyroidism
- Preparation for thyroidectomy in hyperthyroidism
- Therapy prior to and post radio-iodine treatment

CAUTIONS AND CONTRA-INDICATIONS
- Severe blood disorders
- Severe liver impairment (due to prolongation of $t_{1/2}$)
- Pregnancy
- Caution in patients with hypersensitivity to propylthiouracil (cross-sensitivity possible)

SIDE-EFFECTS
- GI disturbance
- Nausea
- Headache
- Fever
- Malaise
- Bone marrow suppression (e.g. agranulocytosis)
- Rash and pruritis
- Myopathy

METABOLISM AND HALF-LIFE   Extensively metabolised in plasma, some in the GI tract and liver during absorption. $t_{1/2}$ is 3–13 h. The majority of administered carbimazole is excreted in the urine as the active metabolite thiamazole.

MONITORING   Monitor for signs and symptoms of bone marrow suppression. FBC should be performed if there is a clinical suspicion of infection. TFTs should be monitored to assess efficacy of treatment.

DRUG INTERACTIONS
- Carbimazole may increase the risk of agranulocytosis when administered with chemotherapy
- Effects of warfarin can be enhanced when taken with carbimazole
- Theophylline levels may be increased with carbimazole

IMPORTANT POINTS
- Due to the risk of agranulocytosis, patients should be warned about the onset of sore throats, bruising or bleeding, fever, malaise and advised to seek medical attention if such symptoms occur
- A gradual reduction in signs and symptoms of thyrotoxicosis is seen over a 3–4 week period
- Carbimazole may be used as a sole agent or as part of a 'block and replace' regimen with levothyroxine
- TFTs and symptoms should guide treatment to render the patient euthyroid

Corticosteroids

EXAMPLES   Prednisolone, hydrocortisone, dexamethasone, methylprednisolone

MECHANISM OF ACTION   Synthetic glucocorticoids that produce the same effects as endogenous cortisol. Glucocorticoids act on intracellular receptors to up-regulate gene transcription. Dexamethasone and prednisolone are approximately 25 and 4 times more potent than hydrocortisone respectively.

INDICATIONS
- Suppression of inflammatory and allergic disorders
- Acute hypersensitivity reactions
- Congenital adrenal hyperplasia
- Cerebral oedema associated with neoplastic disease
- Nausea and vomiting due to chemotherapy

CAUTIONS AND CONTRA-INDICATIONS
- Caution in pregnancy (prolonged or repeated use can increase risk of intra-uterine growth restriction)

SIDE-EFFECTS
- Impaired glucose tolerance
- Osteoporosis
- Proximal myopathy
- Psychiatric reactions (e.g. mood and behavioural changes, insomnia, psychotic symptoms)
- Increased susceptibility to infections
- Hypertension
- Peptic ulceration
- Cushing's syndrome (moon face, truncal obesity, intrascapular fat pad, striae, acne, weight gain)
- Menstrual irregularities
- Bruising and impaired healing
- Ophthalmic effects (e.g. subcapsular cataracts, glaucoma)
- Short stature in children

METABOLISM AND HALF-LIFE   Metabolised predominantly in liver. $t_{1/2}$ is variable (36–54 h for dexamethasone; 12–36 h for prednisolone; 8–12 h for hydrocortisone).

MONITORING   Monitor clinically for adverse effects.

DRUG INTERACTIONS
- Antagonise hypotensive effect of antihypertensives
- Increased risk of peptic ulceration and bleeding with NSAIDs
- Increased risk of hypokalaemia with cardiac glycosides, theophyllines, β_2 agonists and potassium-losing diuretics
- Antagonise hypoglycaemic effect of antidiabetics
- May enhance or reduce anticoagulant effect of warfarin

IMPORTANT POINTS
- Adrenal atrophy results from prolonged corticosteroid use. Therefore, dose of corticosteroid may need to be increased in significant concurrent illness or trauma and abrupt withdrawal (particularly if treatment lasts more than 3 weeks) may result in potentially life-threatening acute adrenal insufficiency
- Corticosteroids exhibit varying mineralocorticoid activity; the mineralocorticoid activity of dexamethasone and betamethasone is negligible and that of prednisolone and methyl-prednisolone is mild

Dipeptidylpeptidase-4 (DDP-4) inhibitors

EXAMPLES   Sitagliptin, vildagliptin

MECHANISM OF ACTION   Blocks the action of the dipeptidylpeptidase-4 enzyme that degrades incretin hormones, including glucagon-like peptide-1 (GLP-1) and glucose-dependent insulinotropic polypeptide (GIP). Incretin hormones increase the synthesis and release of insulin from pancreatic β islet cells when blood glucose concentrations are normal or elevated. Thus DDP-4 inhibitors increase the levels of incretins and subsequently the level of insulin.

INDICATIONS
- Type 2 diabetes mellitus

CAUTIONS AND CONTRA-INDICATIONS
- Diabetic ketoacidosis
- Avoid in pregnancy and breastfeeding

SIDE-EFFECTS
- GI disturbance
- Upper respiratory tract infections
- Peripheral oedema

METABOLISM AND HALF-LIFE $t_{1/2}$ for sitagliptin is ~12–13 h and is excreted predominantly in the urine.

MONITORING   No specific drug monitoring required.

DRUG INTERACTIONS
- DDP-4 inhibitors may cause a small increase in plasma digoxin concentrations.

IMPORTANT POINTS
- NICE guidelines (May 2009) recommend a DDP-4 inhibitor as second-line therapy for patients on either metformin or a sulfonylurea where glycaemic control is inadequate and use of the other class is not appropriate
- A DDP-4 inhibitor may also be considered as third-line therapy

Gonadotrophin-releasing hormone (GnRH) agonists

EXAMPLES   Goserelin, triptorelin

MECHANISM OF ACTION   Synthetic analogues of GnRH cause an initial rise in secretion of gonadotrophins (LH and FSH). Chronic administration causes increased negative feedback, down-regulation of the hypothalamic–pituitary–gonadal axis and a subsequent fall in secretion of gonadal steroids.

INDICATIONS
• Prostate cancer
• Breast cancer (advanced disease or early oestrogen receptor-positive disease)
• Infertility
• Endometriosis (short-term only)
• Induction of endometrial thinning (e.g. in anaemia due to uterine fibroids or prior to surgery)

CAUTIONS AND CONTRA-INDICATIONS
• Pregnancy
• Caution in metabolic bone disease

SIDE-EFFECTS
• Menopausal-like symptoms
• Reduced bone density
• Hypersensitivity reactions
• Headache
• GI disturbance

METABOLISM AND HALF-LIFE $t_{1/2}$ is variable (for goserelin $t_{1/2}$ is 2–4 h); metabolised by hepatic and renal peptidases.

MONITORING   Monitor clinically for tumour 'flare' – initial increase in gonadal steroids may cause transient worsening of signs and symptoms of prostate or breast cancer.

DRUG INTERACTIONS
• Avoid concomitant use of drugs which raise prolactin levels (such agents down-regulate GnRH receptors in the pituitary)

IMPORTANT POINTS
• Anti-androgens (e.g. cyproterone, bicalutamide) are used to inhibit tumour 'flare' before commencing treatment with GnRH agonists (see Anti-androgens, p.102)
• GnRH agonists should not be used in patients with undiagnosed vaginal bleeding due to potential masking of symptoms of underlying endometrial disease

Hormone replacement therapy (HRT)

MECHANISM OF ACTION   Synthetic oestrogens alleviate the symptoms of oestrogen deficiency (including vasomotor symptoms and urogenital atrophy) and may reduce the risk of post-menopausal osteoporosis. Oestrogens alone induce endometrial hyperplasia; combined preparations also containing progestogens may be given to non-hysterectomised women in order to reduce the risk of endometrial malignancy.

INDICATIONS
- Menopausal symptoms
- Osteoporosis prophylaxis (not recommended as first line in women over 50 years)

CAUTIONS AND CONTRA-INDICATIONS
- Pregnancy
- Current or previous recurrent VTE; caution in patients with risk factors for thromboembolism (including antiphospholipid syndrome)
- Breast or ovarian cancer
- Caution in patients at risk of cardiovascular or cerebrovascular disease
- Caution in uterine fibroids (may increase in size due to HRT)

SIDE-EFFECTS
- VTE
- Increased risk of breast, ovarian and endometrial cancers
- Increased risk of ischaemic stroke
- Increased risk of coronary artery disease if combined HRT started >10 years after menopause
- Nausea and vomiting
- Abdominal cramps and bloating
- Weight gain and fluid retention
- Breast tenderness
- Impaired glucose tolerance
- Mood changes
- Altered serum lipid profile

METABOLISM AND HALF-LIFE $t_{1/2}$ highly variable depending upon formulation; metabolised in the liver and excreted in urine.

MONITORING   Full medical history and physical examination should be performed prior to initiation to identify patients at risk of adverse effects. Routine clinical monitoring for side-effects, including advice to attend national cancer screening programmes.

DRUG INTERACTIONS
- Reduced clinical effectiveness if concomitant use of Cytochrome P450 enzyme inducers (e.g. anticonvulsants, rifampicin)

IMPORTANT POINTS
- HRT should not be used in patients with undiagnosed vaginal bleeding due to potential masking of symptoms of underlying endometrial disease
- Choice of HRT is dependent upon risk of adverse effects and individual preference. In non-hysterectomised women progestogens may be given cyclically (for last 12–14 days of cycle) to induce withdrawal bleeding; alternatively, progestogens may be given continuously. Women with a history of endometriosis should use combined preparations even post-hysterectomy due to ectopic endometrial tissue
- Subcutaneous implants are associated with recurrence of vasomotor symptoms at supra-physiological concentrations and prolonged endometrial stimulation after discontinuation

Incretin mimetics

EXAMPLES   Exenatide

MECHANISM OF ACTION   Bind to and activate glucagon-like peptide-1 (GLP-1) receptors, resulting in increased synthesis and secretion of insulin from pancreatic β islet cells. The action of exenatide is glucose-dependent and therefore as plasma glucose levels fall insulin secretion also reduces. In addition, exenatide also suppresses the inappropriate secretion of glucagon as seen in type 2 diabetes.

INDICATIONS
• Type 2 diabetes mellitus

CAUTIONS AND CONTRA-INDICATIONS
• Diabetic ketoacidosis
• Avoid in severe renal impairment
• Avoid in pregnancy and breastfeeding (due to lack of information about safety)

SIDE-EFFECTS
• GI disturbance
• Weight loss (potentially beneficial)
• Hypoglycaemia
• Headache and dizziness
• Injection site reactions
• Antibody formation
• Acute pancreatitis (uncommon)

METABOLISM AND HALF-LIFE $t_{1/2}$ for exenatide is ∼2.4 h and it is excreted predominantly via the renal route.

MONITORING   No specific drug monitoring required.

DRUG INTERACTIONS
• Exenatide may enhance the anticoagulant effect of warfarin

IMPORTANT POINTS
• Exenatide is administered as twice daily SC injections
• NICE guidelines (May 2009) recommend exenatide as a third-line therapy in patients with complications relating to obesity or where treatment with insulin would have significant occupational implications

Insulins

EXAMPLES   Short-acting – insulin aspart (e.g. NovoRapid®), soluble insulin (e.g. Actrapid®); intermediate-acting – isophane insulin (e.g. Insulatard®); long-acting – insulin glargine (e.g. Lantus®), insulin detemir (e.g. Levemir®).

MECHANISM OF ACTION   Exogenous insulin mimics the effects of endogenous insulin; it increases glycogenesis in the liver, adipose tissue and skeletal muscle and it reduces hepatic gluconeogenesis and glycogenolysis. Additional effects include lipogenesis in peripheral tissues, decreased proteolysis and increased uptake of potassium into cells.

INDICATIONS
- Diabetes mellitus
- Emergency management of hyperkalaemia

CAUTIONS AND CONTRA-INDICATIONS
- Hypoglycaemia

SIDE-EFFECTS
- Hypogylcaemia
- Lipohypertrophy at injection sites
- Weight gain

METABOLISM AND HALF-LIFE   Insulin is predominantly metabolised by receptor-mediated degradation. $t_{1/2}$ is ~30 h.

MONITORING   Blood glucose monitoring is required (ideally daily monitoring of capillary glucose via finger prick testing).

DRUG INTERACTIONS
- Hypoglycaemic effect may be enhanced by oral hypoglycaemic agents (e.g. sulfonylureas), alcohol, ACEIs, β blockers and MAOIs
- Corticosteroids reduce the hypoglycaemic effect when given with insulin

IMPORTANT POINTS
- Insulin regimens vary depending on the type of diabetes and glycaemic control, e.g. basal bolus regimen (short-acting insulin with each meal and long-acting insulin overnight) or a mixture of short- and intermediate-acting insulin given twice a day
- Continuous SC insulin pumps are recommended for patients with unpredictable hypogly-caemia or poorly-controlled diabetes despite optimum multiple dosing (NICE July 2008)
- Insulin requirements increase during intercurrent illness, stress, trauma and puberty due to increases in anti-insulin hormone production (including cortisol, growth hormone and sex hormones)
- Insulin cannot be given enterally as it is degraded in the GI tract. Parenteral administration is required, subcutaneously for routine doses or IV if unwell, DKA, HONK or prior to surgery
- Insulin may be required during pregnancy for pre-existing or gestational diabetes. Poor glycaemic control prior to conception can lead to congenital anomalies. Poor control during pregnancy can result in foetal macrosomia and neonatal hypoglycaemia
- Some insulins need to be stored in a refrigerator; if this advice is not followed the insulins may become inactive and this may result in DKA
- Insulin products are now predominantly biosynthetic; previously they were purified from porcine or bovine insulin

Levothyroxine

MECHANISM OF ACTION   Synthetic form of tetraiodothyronine (T_4) that produces the same peripheral effects as the endogenous hormone.

INDICATIONS
- Hypothyroidism
- Diffuse non-toxic goitre

CAUTIONS AND CONTRA-INDICATIONS
- Caution in ischaemic heart disease and hypertension (initiate levothyroxine therapy at a low dose)
- Thyrotoxicosis

SIDE-EFFECTS
- Usually only seen in excessive dosage
- Diarrhoea and vomiting
- Weight loss
- Muscle weakness
- Palpitations and arrhythmias
- Tremor, restlessness, excitability, insomnia
- Heat intolerance

METABOLISM AND HALF-LIFE $t_{1/2}$ is approximately 1 week. Levothyroxine is partially metabolised to triiodothyronine (T_3); it is excreted in the urine and in faeces.

MONITORING   Monitor TFTs

DRUG INTERACTIONS
- Metabolism of levothyroxine is increased by some antiepileptics and barbiturates
- Absorption of levothyroxine is reduced by oral iron supplements, cimetidine and some antacids
- Dose of antidiabetic agents (including insulin) may need to be increased
- Increased anticoagulant effect of warfarin

IMPORTANT POINTS
- Neonatal hypothyroidism requires prompt treatment with levothyroxine to avoid developmental delay
- In patients with panhypopituitarism or predisposition to adrenal insufficiency, corticosteroid therapy should be initiated prior to starting levothyroxine

Propylthiouracil

MECHANISM OF ACTION   Inhibits the conversion of iodide to iodine which thereby interferes with the degradation of thyroglobulin and thereby reduces T_3 and T_4 production.

INDICATIONS
- Hyperthyroidism – long-term treatment or prio to thyroidectomy
- Patients who are hypersensitive to carbimazole

CAUTIONS AND CONTRA-INDICATIONS
- Hypersensitivity

SIDE-EFFECTS
- Hypothyroidism
- GI disturbance
- Leucopenia
- Headache
- Taste disturbance
- Rash
- Liver failure

METABOLISM AND HALF-LIFE   Metabolised in the liver. $t_{1/2}$ is ~2 h.

MONITORING   Monitor TFTs for efficacy of drug.

DRUG INTERACTIONS
- Increased anticoagulant effect of warfarin due to inhibition of vitamin K activity; INR should be monitored prior to surgical procedures

IMPORTANT POINTS
- TFTs and symptoms should guide treatment to render the patient euthyroid
- Both carbimazole and propylthiouracil cross the placenta and can cause hypothyroidism and a goitre in the fetus, hence the lowest dose possible should be given to control maternal symptoms
- Thyroid storm (also known as thyrotoxic crisis) is a life-threatening, hypermetabolic state resulting from excessive release of thyroid hormones. It is a medical emergency and treatment includes hydrocortisone, propanolol and either propylthiouracil or carbimazole

Sulfonylureas

EXAMPLES   Gliclazide, tolbutamide, glibenclamide, glipizide

MECHANISM OF ACTION   Increase the residual capacity of the β cells of the islets of Langerhans to secrete insulin, therefore increasing plasma glucose clearance. Sulfonylureas exert their pharmacodynamic properties by binding to high-affinity receptors on the ATP-sensitive potassium (KATP) channels on β islet cell plasma membranes.

INDICATIONS
• Type 2 diabetes mellitus

CAUTIONS AND CONTRA-INDICATIONS
• Ketoacidosis
• Severe hepatic impairment
• Acute porphyria

SIDE-EFFECTS
• GI disturbance
• Hypoglycaemia
• Blood disorders
• Deranged liver function (e.g. cholestatic jaundice and hepatitis)
• Hypersensitivity reactions (predominantly skin reactions)

METABOLISM AND HALF-LIFE   Variable – e.g. glipizide has a $t_{1/2}$ of ~2–3 h and its metabolism is mainly in the liver to inactive metabolites. $t_{1/2}$ for gliclazide is 10–12 h.

MONITORING   No specific drug monitoring required.

DRUG INTERACTIONS
• Hypoglycaemic effects may be enhanced with warfarin
• Fluconazole increases plasma sulfonylurea levels

IMPORTANT POINTS
• Glibenclamide has a longer half-life hence an increased risk of hypoglycaemia
• Patients should be counselled about the risk of hypoglycaemia and how to recognise and treat it
• Sulfonylureas can cause weight gain and therefore are not first choice in obese patients

Thiazolidinediones

EXAMPLES   Pioglitazone

MECHANISM OF ACTION   PPAR agonists in adipose tissue, skeletal muscle and liver (insulin target tissues). When stimulated, PPAR-γ receptors upregulate transcription to increase production of proteins responsible for glucose transport and utilisation, hence reducing peripheral insulin resistance.

INDICATIONS
• Type 2 diabetes mellitus (single, dual or triple therapy)

CAUTIONS AND CONTRA-INDICATIONS
• Hypersensitivity
• Cardiac failure
• ACS
• Liver disease
• Patients in DKA

SIDE-EFFECTS
• GI disturbance
• Headaches
• Weight gain
• Liver toxicity
• Anaemia
• Dyslipidaemia
• Oedema

METABOLISM AND HALF-LIFE   Predominantly metabolised by the liver, particularly CYP2C8. $t_{1/2}$ for pioglitazone is 5–6 h.

MONITORING   Monitor LFTs prior to commencing and during treatment due to risk of hepatotoxicity.

DRUG INTERACTIONS
• Reduced plasma levels when given with rifampicin, phenytoin, phenobarbital and carbamazepine (inducers of CYP2C8)

IMPORTANT POINTS
• Can be used as monotherapy or in combination with metformin or sulfonylureas
• Treatment should be initiated and monitored by a hospital specialist
• Rosiglitazone is no longer routinely prescribed in the UK due to the associated risk of heart disease

Contraceptives

MECHANISM OF ACTION

COCP – contains both oestrogen and progesterone that act to inhibit the hypothalamo—pituitary axis. Negative feedback on the hypothalamus reduces GnRH secretion and therefore FSH and LH release from the anterior pituitary. The absence of FSH and LH prevent follicular development and ovulation respectively. The absence of ovarian progesterone and oestrogen adversely affect development of the uterine endometrium and result in reduced volume and less viscous cervical secretions.

POP and parenteral (IM) progesterone preparations – have the endometrial and cervical effects as described above but do not inhibit ovulation.

INDICATIONS
- Contraception
- Menstrual symptoms (COCP only)

CAUTIONS AND CONTRA-INDICATIONS
- History of VTE (COCP only)
- History of arterial disease
- Pregnancy
- Liver disease
- History of breast cancer

SIDE-EFFECTS
- Migraine
- Nausea and vomiting
- Changes in body weight
- Hypertension (COCP only)
- Venous thromboembolic disease (COCP only)
- Fluid retention
- Menstrual disturbances (on discontinuation of depot progesterone)

METABOLISM AND HALF-LIFE   Oestrogen (ethinylestradiol) is metabolised in the liver and $t_{1/2}$ is ~36 h. Progesterone is also metabolised in the liver and $t_{1/2}$ varies – $t_{1/2}$ for levonorgestrel is 26 h; $t_{1/2}$ for norethisterone is 7 h.

MONITORING   No specific drug monitoring required.

DRUG INTERACTIONS
- Antimicrobials that induce liver enzymes (e.g. erythromycin, rifampicin) can reduce the efficacy of the hormonal preparations (both oral and IM)
- Antimicrobials that do not induce liver enzymes (e.g. ampicillin, doxycyline) can affect efficacy by altering gut flora that are responsible for recycling of the hormone content
- St John's wort reduces the contraceptive effect of oestrogen and progesterone
- Carbamazepine and phenytoin increase the metabolism of oestrogen and progesterone pills, thereby reducing efficacy

IMPORTANT POINTS
- There is an increased risk of breast and cervical cancer and reduced risk of ovarian and endometrial cancer with use of the COCP
- COCP-induced high BP occurs in 1% of women. It can take up to 4 months for the blood pressure to return to baseline following cessation of the COCP
- Oestrogen-containing contraceptives should be stopped 4 weeks before major or lower limb surgery and recommenced 2 weeks after full mobilisation
- Severe diarrhoea and vomiting can reduce absorption of the drug and, therefore, efficacy. Additional contraceptive measures should be taken for 7 days if the illness lasts more than 24 h

Contraceptives (continued)

- If a pill is missed (i.e. 24 h late), the next pill should be taken as soon as remembered and the rest of the pack continued. If 2 or more pills are missed, then additional contraceptive measures should be taken for 7 days. However, consult the guidelines for different types of hormonal contraception, as preparations vary and the timing during the cycle the pill(s) were missed
- Other types of contraception include barrier methods (condoms, diaphragms, caps), hormone implants, intrauterine devices (copper or hormone-impregnated coils) and transdermal patches

Mifepristone

MECHANISM OF ACTION   Synthetic steroid that antagonises the action of progesterone at progesterone receptors in the uterus (endometrium and myometrium), particularly if primed by prostaglandins, resulting in cervical dilatation and uterine contraction.

INDICATIONS
- Medical termination of intrauterine pregnancy
- Preparation of cervix prior to surgical termination of pregnancy

CAUTIONS AND CONTRA-INDICATIONS
- Uncontrolled severe asthma
- Suspected ectopic pregnancy
- Chronic adrenal failure
- Acute porphyria
- Liver disease
- Renal impairment

SIDE-EFFECTS
- GI cramps
- Uterine contractions
- Vaginal bleeding
- Urticarial rash

METABOLISM AND HALF-LIFE   Metabolised in the liver and excreted in the GI tract; $t_{1/2}$ is ~18 h.

MONITORING   No specific drug monitoring required.

DRUG INTERACTIONS
- Can reduce the efficacy of corticosteroid therapy (including inhaled steroids) for 3–4 days

IMPORTANT POINTS
- A single oral dose of mifepristone is given with a dose of misoprostol (a prostaglandin administered PV (unlicensed indication)) for medical termination of pregnancy
- Women should be warned of potentially severe vaginal blood loss

Oxybutynin

MECHANISM OF ACTION   A competitive antagonist of ACh at post-synaptic muscarinic receptors, resulting in smooth muscle relaxation in the bladder. Oxybutynin exerts its effects by blocking M_2 and M_3 receptors of the bladder and detrusor muscle. In patients with detrusor instability or hyperreflexia this serves to increase bladder capacity.

INDICATIONS
- Urinary frequency, urgency and incontinence
- Neurogenic bladder instability
- Nocturnal enuresis secondary to overactive bladder

CAUTIONS AND CONTRA-INDICATIONS
- Myasthenia gravis
- Urinary retention
- Intestinal obstruction
- Caution in renal and hepatic impairment

SIDE-EFFECTS
- Dry mouth
- Blurred vision
- Constipation
- Dry eyes
- Drowsiness

METABOLISM AND HALF-LIFE   Extensively metabolised by Cytochrome P450 enzymes to inactive metabolites. $t_{1/2}$ is $\sim$13 h.

MONITORING   No specific drug monitoring required.

DRUG INTERACTIONS
- Increased antimuscarinic side-effects when taken with TCAs and sedating antihistamines
- Oxybutynin antagonises the effects of metoclopramide on the GI tract

IMPORTANT POINTS
- Modified release preparations are effective and have a better side-effect profile; they are also more expensive
- Oxybutynin may rarely precipitate acute closed-angle glaucoma
- Oxybutynin may aggravate hyperthyroidism and cardiac failure
- Elderly patients are particularly susceptible to side-effects, with an increased risk of falls
- Solifenacin and tolterodine are other antimuscarinics which act predominantly on the detrusor muscle and may be used for the same indications. Solifenacin and tolterodine are better tolerated than oxybutynin, with fewer adverse effects reported by patients

Oxytocin

MECHANISM OF ACTION   Synthetic form of oxytocin that produces the same effects as the endogenous hormone, which is released from the posterior pituitary gland. Oxytocin acts on specific oxytocin receptors in the myometrium to stimulate smooth muscle contraction.

INDICATIONS
- Induction or augmentation of labour (in conjunction with other agents)
- Incomplete, inevitable or missed abortion
- Prevention of post-partum haemorrhage

CAUTIONS AND CONTRA-INDICATIONS
- Hypertonic uterine contractions
- Any condition in which vaginal delivery is inadvisable (e.g. cephalopelvic disproportion)
- Caution in pre-eclamptic toxaemia (avoid if severe)
- Caution in secondary uterine inertia
- Caution in cardiovascular disease (avoid if severe)
- Caution in patients with history of lower-uterine segment caesarean section
- Caution in women over 35 years

SIDE-EFFECTS
- Nausea and vomiting
- Uterine hyperstimulation (may cause uterine rupture or foetal distress/asphyxia/death)
- Transient hypotension if rapid bolus dose administered
- Fluid retention (if severe, water intoxication and hyponatraemia)
- In overdose, placental abruption and amniotic fluid embolism may occur
- Rarely disseminated intravascular coagulation

METABOLISM AND HALF-LIFE $t_{1/2}$ is ~5 min, hence oxytocin is administered as a continuous intravenous infusion. Oxytocin is metabolised in the liver and excreted via biliary and renal routes.

MONITORING   CTG and clinical monitoring is required. If prolonged use, monitor U&Es.

DRUG INTERACTIONS
- Prostaglandins potentiate the effects of oxytocin, therefore avoid concomitant use
- Oxytoxic effect reduced by inhalation anaesthetics; also enhanced hypotensive effect and increased risk of cardiac arrhythmias with concomitant use
- Increased risk of hypertension with sympathomimetic vasopressors

IMPORTANT POINTS
- An electrolyte-containing diluent should be used (i.e. not dextrose solution) in prolonged oxytocin administration to avoid water intoxication and hyponatraemia
- Oxytocin may be administered intramuscularly with ergometrine (a uterine smooth muscle stimulant) in the prevention and treatment of post-partum haemorrhage
- NICE (July 2008) has produced guidance on the induction of labour
- Recent studies have suggested its potential use in the treatment of shyness (colloquially known as the 'love hormone')

Phosphodiesterase type 5 inhibitors

EXAMPLES   Sildenafil, vardenafil

MECHANISM OF ACTION   Nitric oxide activates guanylyl cyclase to convert GTP to cGMP, which causes smooth muscle relaxation and consequent vasodilatation. These agents prevent degradation of cGMP by phosphodiesterase type 5, thereby potentiating vasodilatation.

INDICATIONS
- Erectile dysfunction
- Pulmonary artery hypertension

CAUTIONS AND CONTRA-INDICATIONS
- ACS
- Recent stroke
- Hypotension (systolic BP <90 mmHg)
- Patients with a history of non-arteritic ischaemic optic neuropathy
- Caution in cardiovascular disease and left ventricular outflow obstruction
- Caution in anatomical deformation of the penis and in patients at risk of priapism (e.g. sickle cell disease, myeloma, leukaemia)

SIDE-EFFECTS
- Headache
- Flushing
- Nasal congestion and epistaxis
- Palpitations
- Hypotension
- Priapism
- GI disturbance (including dysphagia and dyspepsia)
- Visual disturbances (rarely, non-arteritic ischaemic optic neuropathy)
- Cardiovascular events

METABOLISM AND HALF-LIFE   Sildenafil is metabolised in the liver; $t_{1/2}$ is 4–6 h.

MONITORING   Monitor clinically for adverse effects.

DRUG INTERACTIONS
- Concomitant use of nitrate-based medications (e.g. GTN, ISMN), nicorandil and nebivolol may cause potentially life-threatening hypotension
- Enhanced hypotensive effect with antihypertensives
- Plasma concentration of phosphodiesterase type 5 inhibitors is increased by drugs that inhibit CYP3A4 (e.g. cimetidine, erythromycin, itraconazole)

IMPORTANT POINTS
- Phosphodiesterase type 5 inhibitors are administered orally and are, therefore, commonly preferred to intracavernosal agents used in the management of erectile dysfunction (such as prostaglandin E_1)
- These agents are only available to patients in whom erectile dysfunction has occurred as a result of an underlying pathology (e.g. diabetes, multiple sclerosis) or where erectile dysfunction is causing severe distress

Alkylating agents

EXAMPLES Cyclophosphamide, chlorambucil, melphalan, ifosfamide

MECHANISM OF ACTION Cause covalent bonding of an alkyl group to nucleophilic molecules, particularly the purines and pyrimidines of DNA. Alkylation of DNA results in single strand breaks (due to depurination), base pair mismatching or cross-link formation between DNA strands.

INDICATIONS
- Broad spectrum of anti-tumour activity, including haematological malignancies, soft tissue and solid organ tumours
- Rheumatoid arthritis and other autoimmune conditions (cyclophosphamide)

CAUTIONS AND CONTRA-INDICATIONS
- Pregnancy (due to teratogenicity)
- Caution in hepatic or renal impairment (dose reduction may be required)

SIDE-EFFECTS
- Nausea and vomiting
- Myelosuppression (e.g. increased risk of neutropenic sepsis, anaemia and thrombocytopenia)
- Tumour lysis syndrome and hyperuricaemia
- Skin hyperpigmentation and alopecia
- Hypersensitivity reactions (including Stevens–Johnson syndrome)
- Urothelial damage (rarely haemorrhagic cystitis)
- Interstitial pneumonitis and pulmonary fibrosis (melphalan)
- Long-term risk of leukaemia and carcinogenesis

METABOLISM AND HALF-LIFE Variable – e.g. cyclophosphamide and chlorambucil require hepatic activation ($t_{1/2}$ is 3–12 h and ~1.3 h respectively); melphalan degrades spontaneously ($t_{1/2}$ is ~1.5 h).

MONITORING FBC should be checked before each treatment; FBC and U&Es should be monitored regularly.

DRUG INTERACTIONS
- Vaccination with live-organism vaccines are not recommended in patients on immuno-suppressants
- Risk of hypoglycaemia in concomitant use of cyclophosphamide and oral hypoglycaemic drugs

IMPORTANT POINTS
- Drug combinations and dosing regimens are complex therefore chemotherapeutic agents should only be used by specialists
- Resistance to alkylating drugs may occur; causes include reduced membrane transport and inactivation of the agents by hydroxylation
- Mesna can be used in combination with cyclophosphamide or ifosfamide to reduce the risk of haemorrhagic cystitis

Anthracyclines

EXAMPLES Doxorubicin, daunorubicin, epirubicin, idarubicin

MECHANISM OF ACTION Anthracyclines intercalate between nucleic acid base pairs within DNA molecules, interfering with DNA replication and transcription. They also inhibit topoisomerase II, which prevents ligation of DNA strand breaks. These combined effects result in cell death.

INDICATIONS
- Broad spectrum of anti-tumour activity, including haematological malignancies and some solid organ tumours

CAUTIONS AND CONTRA-INDICATIONS
- Severe liver disease
- Recent MI/arrhythmias
- Heart failure
- Pregnancy
- Breastfeeding
- Caution in elderly and patients with hypertension or a history of cardiac disease

SIDE-EFFECTS
- GI disturbance
- Hyperpigmentation of skin, nails and mucous membranes (epirubicin)
- Myelosuppression
- Rarely SVT
- Red discolouration of urine
- Heart failure (doxorubicin)
- Oral mucositis
- Alopecia

METABOLISM AND HALF-LIFE $t_{1/2}$ for doxorubicin is 55 h; $t_{1/2}$ for epirubicin is 40 h.

MONITORING ECG should be performed prior to commencing treatment; regular ECG monitoring should be undertaken during the course of therapy.

DRUG INTERACTIONS
- Increased risk of cardiotoxicity when anthracyclines are given with trastuzumab

IMPORTANT POINTS
- Drug combinations and dosing regimens are complex therefore chemotherapeutic agents should only be used by specialists
- Anthracyclines can lead to the generation of free radical compounds that cause the peroxidation of cardiac sarcoplasmic reticulum; this may result in necrosis of the myocardium. Epirubicin is the least cardiotoxic agent in this group
- Extravasation of anthracyclines can cause severe tissue necrosis

Anti-androgens

EXAMPLES Cyproterone acetate, flutamide, bicalutamide

MECHANISM OF ACTION Blocks dihydrotestosterone receptors in peripheral tissues, including the prostate gland. Negative feedback on the hypothalamo–pituitary axis reduces LH release, which in turn decreases testicular testosterone release.

INDICATIONS
- Prostate cancer
- Acne and hirsutism in women (cyproterone)
- Severe hypersexuality and sexual deviation in men (cyproterone)

CAUTIONS AND CONTRA-INDICATIONS
- Liver disease
- Severe diabetes
- Sickle cell anaemia
- Severe depression
- Malignant disease
- Previous thromboembolic disease
- N.B. None of the above are contraindications if being used for prostate cancer

SIDE-EFFECTS
- Hepatotoxicity
- Changes in weight and hair distribution
- Fatigue
- Dyspnoea
- Gynaecomastia

METABOLISM AND HALF-LIFE Metabolised by pathways in the liver (particularly CYP3A4 enzyme) and excreted via biliary and renal routes. $t_{1/2}$ is ~2 days.

MONITORING Monitor FBC, LFTs and adrenocortical function periodically.

DRUG INTERACTIONS
- Reduced doses of thiazolidinediones may be needed as their hepatic metabolism is inhibited by cyproterone acetate
- There is an increased risk of statin-associated myopathy and rhabdomyolysis for similar reasons

IMPORTANT POINTS
- Anti-androgens antagonise the flare in testosterone production associated with gonadorelin therapy; anti-androgens should be given 3 days prior to the initiation of treatment with gonadorelin analogues and continued for 3 weeks (see Gonadotrophin-releasing hormone (GnRH) agonists, p.86)
- Can be used as palliative treatment when gonadorelins or orchidectomy are contraindicated
- Cyproterone acetate can be used to treat acne and hirsutism in women with PCOS, where these symptoms are due to elevated testosterone levels

Antimetabolites

EXAMPLES   Mercaptopurine, cytarabine, capecitabine, fluorouracil, methotrexate

MECHANISM OF ACTION   Antimetabolites directly or indirectly interfere with DNA and RNA molecules and enzymes thereby inhibiting cell division. Mercaptopurine is a purine analogue; cytarabine impedes pyrimidine synthesis; and capecitabine is metabolised to fluorouracil, which specifically inhibits thymidine synthesis (see also Methotrexate, p.113).

INDICATIONS
- Broad spectrum of antitumour activity, including haematological malignancies, soft tissue and solid organ tumours
- Rheumatoid arthritis and other autoimmune conditions (methotrexate)

CAUTIONS AND CONTRA-INDICATIONS
- Pregnancy
- Breastfeeding
- Caution in hepatic or renal impairment

SIDE-EFFECTS
- Myelosuppression
- Nausea and vomiting
- Alopecia
- Oral mucositis
- Tumour lysis syndrome and hyperuricaemia

METABOLISM AND HALF-LIFE   Extensively metabolised in the liver. $t_{1/2}$ for mercaptopurine is 1–2 h; $t_{1/2}$ for cytarabine is $\sim$10 min; $t_{1/2}$ for capecitabine is $\sim$45 min; $t_{1/2}$ for fluorouracil is 10–20 min.

MONITORING   Monitor FBC due to risk of myelosuppression. Monitor LFTs and renal function in patients with pre-existing liver or kidney disease.

DRUG INTERACTIONS
- Avoid using allopurinol with capecitabine as it reduces its efficacy
- Increased risk of mercaptopurine toxicity when given with allopurinol
- Fluorouracil inhibits the metabolism of phenytoin, thereby increasing serum levels

IMPORTANT POINTS
- Drug combinations and dosing regimens are complex therefore chemotherapeutic agents should only be used by specialists
- Antimetabolites are teratogenic but are not associated with a long-term risk of leukaemias

Antiproliferative immunosuppressants

EXAMPLES Azathioprine, mycophenolate

MECHANISM OF ACTION Azathioprine is metabolised to 6-mercaptopurine, which enters cells and is then converted to purine analogues. These are incorporated into replicating DNA and also inhibit *de novo* purine synthesis, hence reducing immune cell division. Mycophenolate is metabolised to mycophenolic acid, which reversibly inhibits the synthesis of guanosine. T- and B-lymphocytes are dependent on *de novo* synthesis of purines whereas other cell types can utilise salvage pathways hence antiproliferative immunosuppressants have more potent cytostatic effects on lymphocytes than on other cells.

INDICATIONS
- Inflammatory bowel disease (azathioprine)
- Organ transplant recipients (azathioprine and mycophenolate)
- Rheumatoid arthritis (azathioprine)
- Autoimmune conditions (including SLE, haemolytic anaemia) (azathioprine)

CAUTIONS AND CONTRA-INDICATIONS
- Hypersensitivity to mercaptopurine (azathioprine)
- Pregnancy and breastfeeding

SIDE-EFFECTS
- Bone marrow suppression
- Increased susceptibility to infection
- GI disturbance
- GI ulceration (mycophenolate)
- Increased risk of malignancies, especially skin
- Liver disease/cholestatic jaundice
- Hair loss

METABOLISM AND HALF-LIFE 6-mercaptopurine is metabolised by xanthine oxidase prior to excretion in urine; $t_{1/2}$ for 6-mercaptopurine is 1–3 h. Mycophenolic acid is metabolised by glucuronyl transferase prior to excretion in urine; $t_{1/2}$ for mycophenolic acid is ~18 h.

MONITORING Monitor FBC regularly due to risk of bone marrow suppression.

DRUG INTERACTIONS
- Increased risk of haematological toxicity if given with co-trimoxazole
- Reduced doses of azathioprine should be given if also taking allopurinol (xanthine oxidase inhibitor)

IMPORTANT POINTS
- Azathioprine is a steroid-sparing agent and can be used as monotherapy or in combination with corticosteroids to produce immunosuppressant effects
- Mycophenolate is used in combination with ciclosporin and corticosteroids for the prophylaxis of acute rejection in renal, hepatic and cardiac transplantation
- In the management of chronic disease therapeutic effects may take weeks or months to become apparent

Calcineurin inhibitors

EXAMPLES   Ciclosporin, tacrolimus

MECHANISM OF ACTION   Bind to and inhibit calcineurin phosphatase thereby blocking activation of downstream transcription factors that regulate T-lymphocyte activation.

INDICATIONS
- Prevention of transplant graft rejection
- Rheumatoid arthritis
- Treatment and prophylaxis of graft-versus-host disease
- Psoriasis

CAUTIONS AND CONTRA-INDICATIONS
- Caution in renal and hepatic impairment (may require dose adjustment)
- Caution in hyperuricaemia (may be exacerbated by ciclosporin)
- Avoid concomitant use of ciclosporin and tacrolimus

SIDE-EFFECTS
- Nephrotoxicity (dose-dependent rise in serum urea and creatinine initially)
- Hypertension
- Hepatic dysfunction
- GI disturbance
- Hyperlipidaemia
- Hirsutism and gingival hypertrophy
- Hypomagnesaemia
- Increased risk of lymphomas, skin and other tumours
- Increased susceptibility to infections
- Cardio- and neuro-toxicity (tacrolimus)

METABOLISM AND HALF-LIFE   Eliminated predominantly via the biliary route; $t_{1/2}$ for ciclosporin is $\sim$19 h and $t_{1/2}$ for tacrolimus is 43 h (reduced to 12–16 h in transplant recipients due to increased clearance rates resulting from increased unbound fraction or corticosteroid induced metabolism).

MONITORING   Monitor U&Es (including magnesium), LFTs and lipid profile. Monitor BP (may require treatment with antihypertensives) and ECG (particularly QTc). Echocardiography is advised for patients on tacrolimus therapy.

DRUG INTERACTIONS
- Increased risk of hyperkalaemia with ACEIs, ARBs and potassium-sparing diuretics
- Increased nephrotoxicity with NSAIDs and aminoglycosides
- Plasma concentration of calcineurin inhibitors are increased by macrolides, CCBs and grapefruit juice
- Plasma concentration of calcineurin inhibitors are reduced by anticonvulsants
- Risk of myopathy with rosuvastatin increased by concomitant use of ciclosporin
- Risk of digoxin toxicity increased by concomitant use of ciclosporin

IMPORTANT POINTS
- Patients taking ciclosporin should be advised to avoid excess exposure to ultraviolet light
- Patients should be warned of possible immediate and delayed adverse effects of calcineurin inhibitors

Other antineoplastic drugs

MECHANISM OF ACTION
Platinum compounds (e.g. carboplatin, cisplatin) – inhibit DNA synthesis by creating intra- and interstrand cross links.

Taxanes (e.g. docetaxel, paclitaxel) – bind to tubulin and disrupt the microtubular network that is necessary for mitosis.

INDICATIONS
- Broad spectrum of anti-tumour activity (platinum compounds)
- Breast and ovarian tumours (taxanes)

CAUTIONS AND CONTRA-INDICATIONS
- Pregnancy and breastfeeding
- Caution in renal and hepatic impairment

SIDE-EFFECTS
- Nausea and vomiting
- Myelosuppression (e.g. increased risk of neutropenic sepsis, anaemia and thrombocytopenia)
- Tumour lysis syndrome and hyperuricaemia
- Peripheral neuropathy
- Hypersensitivity reactions (especially taxanes)
- Renal toxicity (platinum compounds)
- Ototoxicity (platinum compounds)
- Cardiac conduction defects and arrhythmias (taxanes)

METABOLISM AND HALF-LIFE   Metabolism, elimination and $t_{1/2}$ vary within and between classes.

MONITORING   FBC and U&Es should be monitored regularly.

DRUG INTERACTIONS
- Increased risk of nephro- and ototoxicity if platinum compounds used with diuretics
- Increased risk of pulmonary toxicity if anthracyclines given with platinum compounds
- Taxanes reduce absorption of digoxin and phenytoin

IMPORTANT POINTS
- Drug combinations and dosing regimens are complex therefore chemotherapeutic agents should only be used by specialists
- Hypersensitivity reactions associated with taxanes may be avoided by premedication with a corticosteroid, an antihistamine and a histamine H_2 receptor antagonist

Selective oestrogen receptor modulators (SERMs)

MECHANISM OF ACTION

Tamoxifen – competitive oestrogen receptor antagonist that reduces cell division in oestrogen-dependent tissues (e.g. breast). Tamoxifen has partial agonist effects on the endometrium, the urogenital epithelium, bone remodelling and cholesterol metabolism.

Aromatase inhibitors (e.g. anastrozole, exemestane) – inhibit the peripheral conversion of androgens to oestrogens by the aromatase enzyme complex.

Raloxifene – oestrogen receptor agonist with predominant effects on bone remodelling and lipid metabolism.

Clomifene – oestrogen receptor antagonist that acts in the hypothalamus to inhibit negative feedback, resulting in a rise in GnRH and subsequent increases in FSH and LH. This promotes follicular development and ovulation.

INDICATIONS
- Breast cancer (tamoxifen and aromatase inhibitors)
- Anovulatory infertility (clomifene)
- Postmenopausal osteoporosis (raloxifene)

CAUTIONS AND CONTRA-INDICATIONS
- Pregnancy
- Caution in patients with risk factors for VTE
- Caution in renal and hepatic impairment

SIDE-EFFECTS
- Menopausal symptoms (oedema, hot flushes and urogenital atrophy)
- GI disturbance
- VTE (tamoxifen)
- Endometrial changes including cancer (tamoxifen)
- Osteoporosis (aromatase inhibitors)

METABOLISM AND HALF-LIFE Extensive hepatic metabolism; long $t_{1/2}$ (1–7 days).

MONITORING Monitor clinically for adverse effects.

DRUG INTERACTIONS
- Enhanced anticoagulant effect of warfarin
- Absorption of raloxifene reduced by colestyramine

IMPORTANT POINTS
- Aromatase inhibitors do not inhibit gonadal oestrogen synthesis and therefore are ineffective in pre-menopausal women
- SERMs should not be used in patients with undiagnosed vaginal bleeding due to potential masking of symptoms of underlying endometrial disease
- Due to the risk of ovarian cancer, clomifene should not be given for more than 6 cycles

Trastuzumab (Herceptin®)

MECHANISM OF ACTION This is a recombinant IgG monoclonal antibody against HER2, a tyrosine kinase receptor. Binding of trastuzumab inhibits downstream signalling and ultimately serves to promote cell cycle arrest and apoptosis.

INDICATIONS
- Early HER2-positive breast cancer
- Metastatic HER2-positive breast cancer
- Metastatic HER2-positive gastric cancer

CAUTIONS AND CONTRA-INDICATIONS
- Severe dyspnoea at rest
- Caution in patients with cardiac risk factors

SIDE-EFFECTS
- Cardiotoxicity (including heart failure, hypertension, hypotension, palpitations, arrythmias and cardiomyopathy)
- Hypersensitivity reactions
- Headache and dizziness
- Wheezing and dyspnoea; rarely life-threatening pulmonary events
- GI disturbance

METABOLISM AND HALF-LIFE Trastuzumab is cleared via the reticuloendothelial system; $t_{1/2}$ is 28–38 days.

MONITORING All patients should undergo cardiac assessment (including history, physical examination, ECG and cardiac imaging) prior to initiating treatment and on a regular basis (at least every 3 months).

DRUG INTERACTIONS
- Concomitant use of anthracyclines increases risk of cardiotoxicity

IMPORTANT POINTS
- Only 25–30% of primary breast cancers show over-expression of HER2
- NICE has produced more detailed guidance on the indications for trastuzumab therapy
- Administered by IV infusion; resuscitation facilities should be available during treatment

Vinca alkaloids

EXAMPLES   Vinblastine, vincristine

MECHANISM OF ACTION   Bind to tubulin, thereby inhibiting microtubule assembly. This causes arrest of mitosis during metaphase.

INDICATIONS
- Haematological malignancies
- Some solid organ tumours (e.g. breast and lung)

CAUTIONS AND CONTRA-INDICATIONS
- Pregnancy
- Caution in renal and hepatic impairment
- Caution in neuromuscular disease
- Intra-thecal injection is contra-indicated (neurotoxicity is usually fatal)

SIDE-EFFECTS
- Neurotoxicity including sensory, motor and autonomic neuropathies (e.g. paraesthesia, constipation, paresis, areflexia)
- Nausea and vomiting
- Severe local irritation
- Reversible alopecia
- Leucopenia
- Tumour lysis syndrome and hyperuricaemia
- Rarely syndrome of inappropriate ADH secretion

METABOLISM AND HALF-LIFE   Metabolised in the liver and excreted predominantly via biliary route. $t_{1/2}$ for vincristine is 15–155 h hence usually dosed once weekly; $t_{1/2}$ for vinblastine is ~25 h.

MONITORING   FBC should be checked before each treatment; FBC and U&Es should be monitored regularly.

DRUG INTERACTIONS
- Increased neurotoxicity with other drugs acting on the peripheral nervous system
- Serum levels of anticonvulsants and digoxin may be reduced
- Increased risk of myelosuppression with allopurinol, clozapine and isoniazid

IMPORTANT POINTS
- Oral bioavailability is poor therefore administered only via IV route
- Resistance may occur by means of mutations in the binding sites of tubulin
- Vincristine is the most neurotoxic vinca alkaloid; vinblastine has the most myelotoxic effects

Allopurinol

MECHANISM OF ACTION   Competitive inhibitor of xanthine oxidase, preventing the oxidation of xanthine (derived from purine catabolism) to uric acid.

INDICATIONS
- Prophylaxis of gout and of uric acid and calcium oxalate renal calculi
- Prophylaxis of hyperuricaemia associated with cytotoxic drugs

CAUTIONS AND CONTRA-INDICATIONS
- Acute gout
- Caution in renal and hepatic impairment

SIDE-EFFECTS
- Rash and hypersensitivity reactions
- GI disturbance
- Rarely hepatotoxicity or blood disorders

METABOLISM AND HALF-LIFE $t_{1/2}$ is 1–2 h. Allopurinol is eliminated predominantly by conversion to oxipurinol by xanthine oxidase.

MONITORING   No specific drug monitoring required.

DRUG INTERACTIONS
- Increased risk of toxicity with ACEIs
- Increased risk of rash or hypersensitivity reaction with concomitant use of ampicillin, amoxicillin or thiazide diuretics
- Enhanced anticoagulant effect of warfarin
- Allopurinol enhances the effects of azathioprine and mercaptopurine, thereby increasing toxicity

IMPORTANT POINTS
- Allopurinol may prolong episode of acute gout if treatment is initiated during an acute attack; initiate about 1–2 weeks after the acute symptoms have subsided
- If an episode of acute gout occurs during allopurinol therapy, treatment should be continued and the acute attack treated with colchicine or a NSAID (e.g. diclofenac, indometacin, naproxen)
- Other agents that may be used in the long-term management of gout include sulfinpyrazone (either alone or in combination with allopurinol in resistant cases) and probenecid

Aminosalicylic acid compounds (ASAs)

EXAMPLES   Sulfasalazine, mesalazine, balsalazide, olsalazine

MECHANISM OF ACTION   The therapeutic effect of ASA compounds is due to the metabolic breakdown products 5-aminosalicylic acid (5-ASA) and sulfapyridine. Their anti-inflammatory and immunomodulatory effect is mediated by inhibition of prostaglandin and leukotriene production, as well as scavenging reactive oxygen species produced in the bowel.

INDICATIONS
- Ulcerative colitis (induction and maintenance)
- Crohn's disease (active disease)
- Rheumatoid arthritis

CAUTIONS AND CONTRA-INDICATIONS
- Salicylate hypersensitivity
- G6PD deficiency (sulfasalazine)

SIDE-EFFECTS
- GI disturbance
- Headache
- Pancreatitis
- Hepatitis
- Blood disorders (aplastic anaemia, leucopenia, thrombocytopenia)
- Myocarditis/pericarditis

METABOLISM AND HALF-LIFE   ASAs are metabolised in the liver and intestinal mucosa. Variable $t_{1/2}$ dependent on drug. $t_{1/2}$ sulfasalazine is 5–10 h; $t_{1/2}$ mesalazine is ~5 h.

MONITORING   Monitor FBC, U&Es and LFTs prior to initiating treatment and then monthly for the first 3 months due to risk of haematological, renal and hepatic toxicity.

DRUG INTERACTIONS
- Increased risk of leucopenia when given with azathioprine and mercaptopurine

IMPORTANT POINTS
- Patients should be informed of the risk of haematological side-effects and advised to seek medical attention if they develop fevers, sore throat, malaise or unexplained bruising, bleeding or purpura
- ASAs may be given PO or PR (as enemas or suppositories for distal bowel disease)

Colchicine

MECHANISM OF ACTION   The precise mechanism is not known. Colchicine may inhibit the migration of granulocytes into inflamed areas by impairing microtubule function. This reduces the release of pro-inflammatory enzymes and cytokines, thereby disrupting the inflammatory response.

INDICATIONS
- Acute gout
- Short-term prophylaxis during initiation of therapy with allopurinol (low dose)

CAUTIONS AND CONTRA-INDICATIONS
- Pregnancy
- Caution in renal and hepatic impairment

SIDE-EFFECTS
- GI disturbance (including nausea, vomiting, abdominal pain and diarrhoea)
- Myelosuppression, myopathy and peripheral neuropathy may occur with prolonged treatment

METABOLISM AND HALF-LIFE   Excreted largely unchanged via the biliary route; $t_{1/2}$ is ~10 h.

MONITORING   No specific drug monitoring required.

DRUG INTERACTIONS
- Increased risk of toxicity with macrolides and ciclosporin

IMPORTANT POINTS
- Colchicine is as effective as NSAIDs in the management of acute gout. It is preferable in patients with heart failure and on anticoagulants because colchicine does not cause fluid retention and the risk of GI bleeding is small
- Corticosteroid therapy (prednisolone) is an alternative to colchicine and NSAIDs

Methotrexate

MECHANISM OF ACTION   Competitively inhibits dihydrofolate reductase, which catalyses the conversion of dihydrofolate to tetrahydrofolate. Tetrahydrofolate is a co-factor in thymidine and purine synthesis, therefore methotrexate prevents DNA and RNA synthesis.

INDICATIONS

- Rheumatoid arthritis
- Crohn's disease
- Psoriasis
- Malignant disease (particularly acute lymphoblastic leukaemia)

CAUTIONS AND CONTRA-INDICATIONS

- Hepatic impairment
- Pregnancy (including 3 months prior to conception) and breastfeeding
- Active infection or immunodeficiency syndromes
- Extreme caution in blood disorders
- Caution in ulcerative diseases of the GI tract (e.g. ulcerative colitis, peptic ulceration, ulcerative stomatitis)
- Caution in renal impairment

6 – 12 wks for effect

SIDE-EFFECTS

- Myelosuppression (including leucopenia and neutropenia)
- Hepatotoxicity
- Mucositis (may manifest as GI ulceration)
- Pulmonary fibrosis and pneumonitis
- Rarely pericarditis and pericardial tamponade
- Headaches, drowsiness and blurred vision

METABOLISM AND HALF-LIFE   Unchanged drug is excreted in the urine; $t_{1/2}$ is 3–10 h following low-dose treatment and 8–15 h following high-dose treatment.

MONITORING   FBC, U&Es and LFTs should be checked before initiating treatment. These parameters should initially be monitored weekly and then every 2–3 months when stable. Patients should be advised to monitor for and report any adverse effects, especially sore throat.

DRUG INTERACTIONS

- Increased risk of pulmonary toxicity with cisplatin
- Increased risk of haematological toxicity with corticosteroids and clozapine
- Salicylates and phenytoin increase toxicity via reduced binding to serum albumin
- Penicillins and NSAIDs reduce renal clearance and therefore increase toxicity
- Methotrexate reduces the absorption of digoxin
- Concomitant use of live vaccines should be avoided due to potentially severe or fatal infections

IMPORTANT POINTS

- Patients with a significant pleural effusion or ascites should have these drained prior to treatment with methotrexate because it may accumulate in these fluids, causing myelosuppression on its return to the circulation
- Methotrexate is dosed once weekly; folic acid is routinely co-prescribed to reduce adverse side effects

Antiglaucoma drugs

MECHANISM OF ACTION

β blockers (e.g. timolol) – inhibit rate of production of aqueous humour.

Prostaglandin analogues (e.g. latanoprost) – reduce intraocular pressure by increasing flow via uveoscleral pathway.

Sympathomimetics (e.g. brimonidine) – increase outflow through the trabecular meshwork and reduce aqueous humour production.

Carbonic anhydrase inhibitors (e.g. acetozolamide, dorzolamide) – reduce production of aqueous humour.

Miotics (e.g. pilocarpine) – cause pupillary constriction thereby opening the poorly draining trabecular meshwork.

INDICATIONS
- Primary open-angle glaucoma
- Acute closed-angle glaucoma

CAUTIONS AND CONTRA-INDICATIONS
- β blockers in patients with bradycardia, heart block or uncontrolled heart failure due to systemic absorption of the drug
- Sympathomimetics should be used with caution in patients at risk of acute closed-angle glaucoma due to mydriasis
- Carbonic anhydrase inhibitors should be avoided in hypokalaemia and hyponatraemia
- Miotics should be avoided in acute iritis and anterior uveitis

SIDE-EFFECTS
- Brown pigmentation of iris and blepharitis (prostaglandin analogues)
- Ciliary spasm with headaches, ocular burning and itching (miotics)
- See also β blockers, p.16

METABOLISM AND HALF-LIFE $t_{1/2}$ varies. Topically administered drugs are absorbed through the cornea and predominantly metabolised in the liver.

MONITORING   If carbonic anhydrase inhibitors are used long term, FBC and U&Es should be monitored.

DRUG INTERACTIONS
- β blockers should not be used in conjunction with verapamil (due to risk of AV block)

IMPORTANT POINTS
- These agents are often used in combination with the aim of reducing intraocular pressure; β blockers and prostaglandin analogues (alone or in combination) are typically first choice
- Acute closed-angle glaucoma is a medical emergency, requiring urgent referral to an ophthalmologist. Treatment includes IV acetozolamide, 4% pilocarpine, analgesia and anti-emetics
- Systemic side-effects of these drugs should be considered when prescribing

Depolarising neuromuscular blocking agents

EXAMPLES   Suxamethonium (succinylcholine)

MECHANISM OF ACTION   Mimic the action of ACh by binding to nicotinic receptors and causing membrane depolarisation. The absence of the appropriate hydrolysing enzyme (pseudo-cholinesterase) at the neuromuscular junction results in a much longer duration of action. This persistent depolarisation initiates local current circuits that render voltage-sensitive channels inactive at the neuromuscular junction and halts propagation of further action potentials, ensuring muscles remain relaxed.

INDICATIONS
- Neuromuscular blockade in general anaesthesia

CAUTIONS AND CONTRA-INDICATIONS
- Hypersensitivity to neuromuscular blockers
- Personal or family history of malignant hyperthermia
- Cerebral palsy
- Hyperkalaemia
- Trauma and burns (risk of augmenting hyperkalaemia)
- Personal or family history of neuromuscular disease
- Caution in the presence of glaucoma, detached retina or open eye injury (suxamethonium raises intraocular pressure)

SIDE-EFFECTS
- Post-operative myalgia (common with early mobilisation)
- Increased gastric pressure
- Anaphylactic reactions
- Increased intraocular pressure
- Myoglobinaemia

METABOLISM AND HALF-LIFE $t_{1/2}$ of suxamethonium is $\sim$ 4 min. Its metabolism is catalysed by pseudoesterases in plasma and liver.

MONITORING   Continuous cardiorespiratory monitoring. Three-lead ECG and end-tidal CO_2 monitoring are required.

DRUG INTERACTIONS
- Effects of suxamethonium are potentiated with aminoglycosides, clindamycin and vancomycin
- Increased risk of bradycardia and hypotension when propofol is given with suxamethonium

IMPORTANT POINTS
- Suxamethonium is the only agent used within this group of depolarising agents
- Due to their ability to bind to M_2 muscarinic receptors in the SA node, depolarising agents may trigger severe bradycardia (tachycardia can occur with single use)
- Depolarising agents may induce malignant hyperthermia (see Inhalational anaesthetics, p.117)

Etomidate

MECHANISM OF ACTION Short-acting induction agent that exerts its effect through its GABA(A) agonist activity. The exact mechanism is poorly understood.

INDICATIONS
• Induction of anaesthesia

CAUTIONS AND CONTRA-INDICATIONS
• Hypersensitivity to etomidate
• Caution in hepatic impairment (dose reduction may be required)

SIDE-EFFECTS
• Hypersensitivity reactions including anaphylaxis
• Shivering
• Respiratory depression
• Coughing
• Arrhythmias

METABOLISM AND HALF-LIFE Elimination $t_{1/2}$ is ~3–5 h. Metabolism takes place in the liver with the majority of the drug excreted in the urine as metabolites.

MONITORING Continuous cardiorespiratory monitoring is essential. Three-lead ECG and end tidal CO_2 monitoring are required.

DRUG INTERACTIONS
• Sedatives may potentiate the effects of etomidate
• MAOIs should be stopped 2 weeks prior to administering etomidate
• Risk of hypotension when etomidate is administered with antihypertensives

IMPORTANT POINTS
• Etomidate should only be administered by experienced personnel. Full airway support and continuous monitoring must be established prior to giving etomidate
• Excitatory effects, such as involuntary movements, are witnessed at induction and recovery. These can be reduced by pre-dosing with an opioid or benzodiazepine
• Can cause adrenal suppression with a reduction in cortisol and aldosterone levels (which prevents its wider use)
• Etomidate has the advantage of a faster recovery without an 'anaesthetic hangover' in comparison to other induction agents such as thiopental

Inhalational anaesthetics

EXAMPLES   Halothane, isoflurane, sevoflurane

MECHANISM OF ACTION   Inhalational anaesthetics have three main actions: rendering the patient unconscious, loss of pain perception and loss of reflexes. The central effects of GABA-mediated inhibition are potentiated by these drugs. Once reaching a therapeutic level they negatively affect synaptic transmission and the release of excitatory neurotransmitters.

INDICATIONS
- General anaesthesia

CAUTIONS AND CONTRA-INDICATIONS
- Family history of malignant hyperthermia
- Hypersensitivity
- Moderate-severe hepatic impairment
- Raised intracranial pressure
- Severe cardiovascular or pulmonary disease

SIDE-EFFECTS
- Arrhythmias
- Hypotension
- Mucous membrane irritation causing cough and laryngospasm
- Severe hepatotoxicity (halothane)

METABOLISM AND HALF-LIFE   Variable depending on drug. The majority of the new inhalational anaesthetics undergo rapid and extensive pulmonary elimination. Less than 5% of absorbed sevoflurane is metabolised by the liver.

MONITORING   Continuous cardiorespiratory monitoring is essential. Three-lead ECG and end tidal CO_2 monitoring are required.

DRUG INTERACTIONS
- Increased risk of arrhythmias when adrenaline is administered with inhalational anaesthetics
- Use of inhalational anaesthetics with verapamil or antipsychotics can increase the risk of hypotension

IMPORTANT POINTS
- Inhalational anaesthetics are administered as a mixture with oxygen and nitrous oxide
- Halothane is now rarely used in anaesthesia due to its substantial metabolism and the production of hepatotoxic metabolites
- Speed of induction and recovery of anaesthesia is dependent on the solubility of the anaesthetic in blood and fat. The lower the solubility (blood:gas partition co-efficient) the quicker the rate of induction and recovery of an administered anaesthetic
- Inhalational anaesthetics may very rarely precipitate malignant hyperthermia. This is a hypermetabolic state of skeletal muscle that results in pyrexia and increased oxygen demand. Treatment constitutes disconnecting from the machine/circuit immediately, establishing a definitive airway, administering 100% oxygen, cooling the patient down and administering dantrolene

Lidocaine

MECHANISM OF ACTION Lidocaine serves as a local anaesthetic and an anti-arrhythmic. It binds to open Na^+ channels during phase 0 of the action potential, leaving many channels blocked or inactivated, thereby preventing the propagation of further action potentials.

INDICATIONS
- Ventricular arrhythmias
- Local anaesthetic

CAUTIONS AND CONTRA-INDICATIONS (to IV use as an anti-arrhythmic)
- AV block
- SA disorders
- Severe myocardial depression
- Acute porphyria

SIDE-EFFECTS
- Dizziness
- Paraesthesia
- Drowsiness
- Anaphylaxis
- Hypotension
- Confusion
- Respiratory depression

METABOLISM AND HALF-LIFE Metabolised by the liver to active metabolites. $t_{1/2}$ is 90–120 min when given intravenously. The therapeutic effect of lidocaine, when used as a local anaesthetic, lasts $\sim$2 h.

MONITORING Cardiac monitoring is required when lidocaine is used intravenously. Serum U&Es should be checked for patients on a lidocaine infusion.

DRUG INTERACTIONS
- Increased risk of myocardial depression when lidocaine is given with β blockers or other anti-arrhythmics
- Increased risk of ventricular arrhythmias when lidocaine is given to patients on antipsychotics (due to prolonged QT interval)
- Hepatic clearance of lidocaine maybe delayed when given to patients on cimetidine

IMPORTANT POINTS
- The administration of IV lidocaine warrants continuous ECG monitoring, oxygen and the availability of resuscitation equipment for managing cardiovascular collapse or anaphylaxis
- Lidocaine is a weak base hence its local anaesthetic properties are significantly reduced in acidic environments (e.g. local abscess)
- When used as a local anaesthetic lidocaine may be administered with adrenaline, which causes local vasoconstriction. This results in diminished blood flow and reduced rate of absorption, hence prolonging the effect of lidocaine
- Adrenaline should never be used in the region of end arteries (e.g. fingers, toes, penis) as this may cause ischaemia and consequent tissue necrosis
- The maximum recommended safe dose of lidocaine in local anaesthesia is 3 mg/kg (without adrenaline) and 7 mg/kg (with adrenaline)

Non-depolarising blocking agents

EXAMPLES   Atracurium, pancuronium, vercuronium

MECHANISM OF ACTION   Bind competitively to the α subunit of nicotinic ACh receptors at the neuromuscular junction. This reduces the number of the motor end plate action potentials propagated, resulting in muscle paralysis. Some drugs produce significant autonomic effects due to action at the autonomic ganglia (e.g. hypotension).

INDICATIONS
• Neuromuscular blockade in general anaesthesia

CAUTIONS AND CONTRA-INDICATIONS
• Hypersensitivity to neuromuscular blockers

SIDE-EFFECTS
• Hypotension
• Tachycardia
• Myopathy
• Flushing and bronchospasm (due to histamine release)

METABOLISM AND HALF-LIFE   Variable depending on drug; atracurium is short-acting whereas pancuronium is long-acting. Atracurium has a $t_{1/2}$ of 20 min and hydrolyses spontaneously in plasma. Majority of other non-depolarising blockers are metabolised by the liver.

MONITORING   Continuous cardiorespiratory monitoring. Three-lead ECG and end tidal CO_2 monitoring is required.

DRUG INTERACTIONS
• Inhalational anaesthetics can prolong the effects of atracurium
• Effects of non-depolarising neuromuscular blockers are enhanced by aminoglycosides and clindamycin

IMPORTANT POINTS
• The first muscles to be affected following administration are the eyes. Respiratory muscles are the last to become paralysed and the first to recover
• Anticholinesterase agents should be immediately available for reversal of neuromuscular blockade if necessary
• Dose should be based on ideal body weight (if obese) to avoid excessive dosage

Propofol

MECHANISM OF ACTION   Propofol is an alkyl phenol with short-acting properties and a rapid onset of action. It has been postulated that propofol induces anaesthesia by positively modulating the inhibitory effects of GABA and glycine within the CNS.

INDICATIONS
- Induction of anaesthesia
- Sedation

CAUTIONS AND CONTRA-INDICATIONS
- Hypersensitivity to propofol or its excipients (peanut and soya)

SIDE-EFFECTS
- Burning sensation at site of injection
- Bradycardia
- Hypotension
- Apnoea

METABOLISM AND HALF-LIFE   Elimination $t_{1/2}$ is ~30–60 min, however, the clinical effects last only 2–4 min due to rapid drug redistribution to peripheral tissues from the CNS. Metabolism occurs mainly in the liver with the majority of the drug excreted in the urine.

MONITORING   Continuous cardiorespiratory monitoring is essential. Three-lead ECG and end tidal CO_2 monitoring are required.

DRUG INTERACTIONS
- CNS depressants (e.g. morphine) augment the cardiorespiratory effects of propofol
- Increased risk of bradycardia and hypotension when propofol is given with suxamethonium
- MAOIs should be stopped 2 weeks prior to administering propofol

IMPORTANT POINTS
- Propofol should only be administered by experienced personnel. Full airway support and continuous monitoring must be established prior to drug administration
- Propofol is insoluble in water and therefore formulated as an emulsion, dissolved in soya bean oil emulsified in purified egg phospholipid
- Propofol infusion syndrome is a rare but documented complication associated with long-term sedation with propofol on intensive care. Features include cardiac failure, rhabdomyolysis and renal failure and there is a high associated mortality

Thiopental sodium

MECHANISM OF ACTION   A barbiturate derivative that increases the duration of GABA-dependent Cl^- channel opening in the CNS. This results in hyperpolarisation and inhibition of neuronal activity. The effects appear to be mediated through their interaction with the β subunit within GABA(A) receptors.

INDICATIONS
- Induction of general anaesthesia
- Status epilepticus

CAUTIONS AND CONTRA-INDICATIONS
- Acute porphyria
- Myotonic dystrophy
- Severe cardiovascular disease
- Acute asthma

SIDE-EFFECTS
- Hypotension
- Arrhythmias
- Laryngeal spasm
- Hypothermia
- Anaphylaxis

METABOLISM AND HALF-LIFE   The elimination $t_{1/2}$ is about 11 h. At higher doses the drug exhibits zero-order kinetics. A rapid decline in plasma levels is seen due to rapid redistribution to the brain and kidneys. Further decline in plasma levels are due to hepatic metabolism. Thiopental is strongly bound to plasma proteins that impairs its renal excretion.

MONITORING   Continuous monitoring of cardiorespiratory parameters while on treatment and in the recovery phase. Three-lead ECG and end tidal CO_2 monitoring are essential.

DRUG INTERACTIONS
- Thiopental enhances the hypotensive effects of verapamil
- Enhanced hypotensive effect with β-blockers and antipsychotics
- MAOIs should be stopped 2 weeks before administering thiopental

IMPORTANT POINTS
- Thiopental causes a dose-dependent reduction in cardiac output and TPR which trigger a sympathetic response
- Thiopental is used in the treatment of status epilepticus if no response is seen with benzodiazepines and other anticonvulsants (e.g. phenytoin)
- Following single IV administration rapid induction of anaesthesia is seen with a duration of 5–10 min
- Thiopental sodium may be used as a 'truth serum' (unlicensed use and not recommended!)

Intravenous fluids

CRYSTALLOIDS Crystalloids are solutions that pass freely across the capillary membrane and do not contribute to plasma oncotic pressure. Isotonic crystalloids distribute evenly throughout the interstitial and intravascular spaces.

Examples	Principle constituents		
	Na$^+$ (mmol/l)	Cl$^-$ (mmol/l)	Glucose (g/l)
Normal saline (0.9% NaCl)	154	154	0
5% Dextrose	0	0	50
Dextrose saline (0.18% NaCl 4% Dextrose)	30	30	40
Hartmann's solution (Also contains: K$^+$ 5 mmol/l, Ca^{2+} 2 mmol/l, lactate 29 mmol/l)	131	111	0
Ringer's lactate (Also contains: K$^+$ 4 mmol/l, Ca^{2+} 2.7 mmol/l, lactate 28 mmol/l)	130	109	0

COLLOIDS Colloids are solutions that contain particles that are too large to pass across the capillary membrane and, thus, remain in the intravascular compartment, contributing to the oncotic pressure.

Examples	Principle constituents
5% Albumin	Albumin 50 g/l
Gelatins (e.g. Gelofusine®, Volplex®)	Gelatin polypeptides (variable type and concentration)
Dextrans (e.g. dextran 70)	Polysaccharides (variable type and concentration)

CAUTIONS AND SPECIAL CIRCUMSTANCES
- Sodium chloride solutions are indicated for sodium depletion, whereas sodium chloride and glucose solutions are indicated for sodium and water depletion
- Balanced solutions (e.g. Hartmann's solution or Ringer's lactate) are less likely than 0.9% saline to cause hyperchloraemic acidosis
- Excessive volumes of 5% dextrose or 4%/0.18% dextrose saline solutions should be used with caution due to risk of hyponatraemia
- Colloids may impair normal haemostatic mechanisms, due to non-specific dilutional effects and colloid-specific effects, such as acquired von Willebrand syndrome, inhibition of platelet function and fibrin polymerisation
- Caution should be exercised in patients with evidence of intravascular volume depletion who are oedematous

SIDE-EFFECTS
- Fluid overload
- Electrolyte imbalance
- Hypersensitivity reactions to constituents of colloid solutions

IMPORTANT POINTS

- Fluid prescribing should be directed by maintenance requirements, deficit and ongoing losses
- Maintenance requirements for adults:
    o Na$^+$ 2 mmol/kg/24 h ($\sim$100 mmol)
    o K$^+$ 1 mmol/kg/24 h ($\sim$60 mmol)
    o Water 40 ml/kg/24 h (2.5–3 l)
- Maintenance requirements for children:
    o Electrolytes as per adults
    o Water 100 ml/kg/24 h for first 10 kg of body weight
            50 ml/kg/24 h for next 10 kg of body weight
            25 ml/kg/24 h for additional weight >20 kg
    o e.g. for a 24 kg child = (100 ml $\times$ 10 kg) + (50 ml $\times$ 10 kg) + (25 ml $\times$ 4 kg) = 1600 ml/24 h
- Deficit:
    o This is estimated from clinical features (e.g. dry mucous membranes, reduced skin turgor, sunken facies) and physiological parameters (including pulse, arterial pressure, venous pressure (JVP or CVP), respiratory rate, urine output and capillary refill time)
    o The gold standard for assessing hypovolaemia is flow-based measurements (e.g. trans-oesophageal Doppler, pulse contour analysis) but these are not widely available
- Ongoing losses:
    o Requires charting of losses, for example diarrhoea, vomiting, diuresis and losses from stomas, drains, fistulae and nasogastric aspirates
    o Diarrhoea is relatively rich in K$^+$ and HCO$_3^-$ ions
    o Vomitus is relatively rich in H$^+$, K$^+$ and Cl$^-$ ions
- When the diagnosis of hypovolaemia is in question a bolus of 10–20 ml/kg of colloid or crystalloid should be administered and the patient's clinical response assessed after 15 min; repeated boluses may be required
- Hypovolaemia predominantly due to blood loss should be treated with blood products, however, until these are available a balanced crystalloid or colloid may be used

Blood and transfusion medicine

Blood transfusion is used in a range of conditions from chronic disease to life-threatening emergencies. Blood is centrifuged to produce three main constituents: plasma, platelets and red blood cells.

Blood fraction	Constituents	Blood product
Whole blood	Red blood cells and all plasma constituents	Whole blood
Plasma	Fresh frozen plasma (FFP)	FFP stored at $-30\,°C$ for 24 months
	Clotting factors (factor VIII, von Willebrand factor, fibrinogen)	Cryoprecipitate frozen to $-30\,°C$ within 2 h of preparation
	Albumin	Human albumin solution stored at room temperature
	Immunoglobulins	IV immunoglobulins
Platelets	Platelets	Platelet concentrate which is stored at room temperature for 5 days. 1 unit is obtained from 5 patients
Red bloods cells	Red bloods cells	Red cell concentrate that is stored at $4\,°C$ for 35 days

CAUTIONS AND SPECIAL CIRCUMSTANCES

- Blood transfusions are not without risk, therefore as with any medical treatment, benefit should be weighed up against side-effects
- In order to minimise risks, blood is screened for infections to prevent transmission from donor to recipient. Blood transfusions were a source of hepatitis B and C transmission in people receiving transfusion, in particular prior to the 1990s. Blood is now routinely screened for HIV, hepatitis B and C, syphilis and human T-lymphotropic virus, with additional screening (e.g. for malaria and Chagas disease) if the donor has a travel history
- Other risks include ABO and rhesus incompatibility, hence blood is screened for antibodies to reduce the risk of haemolytic transfusion reactions
- All blood is filtered to remove leucocytes, due to their antigenic potential. Immunocompromised patients require blood products to be irradiated (to remove residual leucocytes and thus avoid graft versus host reactions) and screened for CMV
- Other groups requiring CMV screening include neonates and intrauterine transfusions, pregnant women and HIV-positive patients

SIDE-EFFECTS

- If a patient develops features of a transfusion reaction (including fevers, chills, rigors, tachycardia, hyper- or hypotension, collapse, flushing, urticaria, pain or dyspnoea) the transfusion should be stopped immediately

Tranfusion reaction	Symptoms	Management
Febrile non-haemolytic	Rise in temperature < 1.5 °C	Paracetamol 1 g Continue transfusion slowly
ABO incompatibility:		
• Acute haemolytic	Fever, chills, chest pain, abdominal pain, tachycardia, hypotension, DIC, acute kidney injury	Stop transfusion, return to blood bank with giving set 0.9% saline IV
• Delayed haemolytic	Symptoms occur >24 h after the transfusion	
Mild anaphylactic	Urticaria	Chlorpheniramine 10 mg IV Continue transfusion slowly
Severe anaphylactic	Bronchospasm, angioedema, abdominal pain, hypotension	Stop transfusion, return to blood bank with giving set Chlorpheniramine 10 mg IV Adrenaline 0.5 ml 1:1000 IM
Fluid overload	Dyspnoea, raised CVP	Oxygen Furosemide 40–80 mg IV
Transfusion related acute lung injury (TRALI)	Dyspnoea, frothy haemoptysis, fever, chills, normal CVP	Oxygen Treat as acute respiratory distress syndrome
Iron overload	Weight loss, fatigue, bronze skin, dyspnoea, abdominal pain, arthralgia	Desferrioxamine (iron chelator)
Graft versus host disease	Fever, skin rash, diarrhoea, hepatitis	Immunosuppressive therapy
Immunosuppression	Increased progression of malignancy, transfusion related immunomodulation	
Viral transmission	Symptoms dependent on pathogen	Treatment dependent on pathogen
Post transfusion purpura	Low platelets with bleeding, usually 5–9 days after transfusion	High dose IV immunoglobulins Platelet transfusion
Bacterially contaminated unit	Fever, chills, chest pain, abdominal pain, tachycardia, hypotension	Appropriate antibiotics

IMPORTANT POINTS
- When a patient requires blood products, a blood sample must be sent to the laboratory for the blood group and compatibility to be assessed. This can be done in two ways, depending on the level of urgency

- A 'group and save' sample will establish the ABO group, Rhesus D type and other antibody incompatibility. The blood sample will then be stored for 3–7 days before being destroyed and blood can be made available for the patient within 15–30 min when requested
- A 'crossmatch' sample is needed if a unit of blood product is to be provided immediately. The group and rhesus status is established as well as the compatibility to the unit being provided. In the emergency setting, O negative or type-specific blood can be given while waiting for the crossmatched blood

Index of drugs